We
All
Die
Once

By Dr. Larry Kessler

Table of Contents

Dedication

First and foremost, I would like to thank my wife and children for their patience and understanding throughout the book process. None of this would have been possible without their love and support.

This book is dedicated to my patients and all people who, at one point or another in their lifetimes, will become patients, parents, caregivers and receivers. Only through education and understanding with a sense of reasonability, tolerance and responsibility can we make our health system work for us.

Chapter One: We All Die Once

A lot of what I have to say involves death. We all die. Some of us do it suddenly, some of us spend most of our lives dying. We die violently, quietly, or in the chaos of attempts to save us. We think of death in terms of science, medicine, philosophy, religion and public policy. Every faith and culture has its own death rituals. Some mourn for a lifetime. Some utter a prayer and move on.

I want to tell you some difficult things about modern medicine. Much of what I have to say comes from my experience as a physician working in emergency docks and emergency rooms. I have spent my career in the world of emergency medicine, where death is a constant presence. I see how people die, then I see how their loved ones react. Many of those reactions reveal ways that we are hamstrung by death, leaving us with only tragic options. But other people react differently. Some cultures see the necessity of death, and some individuals have an instinctive ability to regard death as a completion of a life. If the life was well-lived, their grief is tempered by an astounding joy.

Though much of what's here will be connected with death, my main concern is life. The purpose of medicine is to contribute to peoples' happiness by keeping them alive and healthy. When its practitioners have accomplished this, modern medicine has done its job. When we get sidetracked by survival, and forget good health and happiness, we've gone astray. I want to show how American medicine has wandered off the track, often losing sight of its most noble goals. I will also suggest some things we—doctors and patients—can do to steer our medical system back onto the road to better health.

I will be writing about the medicine that keeps many of us alive, but to understand that fully, we must also look at the medical world's efforts to deal with death. We regard death as an evil. Most medical processes are shaped by this attitude. I say it's not that simple. To prove it, let me tell you three very different emergency medicine stories, each about death and those left behind:

Stoic

It was one of those nights. If the ER had been an all-night diner it would've been the kind of shift where the staff couldn't clear a table before the next people sat down to eat. That's fine in a diner, where most problems can be solved with coffee and a sandwich. It's different when your customers are injured, sick or dying.

I'd arrived as several crises loomed, and I wasn't even out of my street clothes when I pulled the curtain to find an elderly Asian woman lying on the cart. Her triage report read: "elderly fall, no further information d\t language barrier." Next to her stood a man whom I took to be her husband. He was holding her hand. He bowed his head slightly, acknowledging my presence with a quality of respect that seems almost odd in western cultures.

I smiled, automatically extending my hand, and introducing myself as the doctor. My hand met air, and my arm fell to my side. The man nodded and smiled, revealing a paucity of stained teeth.

"Okay," I said softly, "what happened here?"

Again he smiled, his eyes revealing polite resignation. He bowed his head once more. With that I understood that I'd just received all he could give me about the history of the case. He couldn't speak English, yet he'd told me things. I could see the bond between them. Seeing it, I realized that, whatever had happened, these two would endure it together. That was a lot to convey when you consider that his communication tools did not include words.

I turned to my patient, and again introduced myself. Again, it wasn't words that mattered. She understood who I was and why I was there. The sounds I was making merely acknowledged it. Her bright eyes and her smile told me she wanted resolution as much as I did. From that I assumed she would be a cooperative patient. That would help a lot in overcoming the language barrier, and dealing with her ailment, whatever it might be.

Like me, my patient was still wearing street clothes. That meant that she hadn't received any attention from a nurse, tech, or aide. She hadn't been prepped in any way beyond being put on the cart. I continued with my assessment with as much speed and thoroughness as possible. Neither patient nor husband flinched as I put on gloves to begin my examination.

She lay motionless as I examined her heart and lungs, which showed no abnormality, then I palpated her head, torso and abdomen. I passively lifted her arms to assess her range of motion without discomfort. As I compressed her hips, she winced and closed her eyes. I'd been halfway expecting this "ah ha" moment. To preserve her dignity I lifted the sheet, forming a wall of privacy. I saw that her left leg was not parallel to her right. With her shoes off I could easily discern her left toes pointing outward, the left being shorter than the right. Classic hip fracture, I surmised. I completed the assessment with a quick squeeze of her knees. This might show any related injury. There wasn't any.

As I finished this initial examination, I turned to the couple to explain, then remembered that my words would be useless. I communicated as best I could, hoping they might catch the general idea from my tone. Finally I stepped out, and wrote orders for x-rays, a consultant, and admission for surgery. I finished, glad to have had at least one easy case on a night that promised to be chaotic.

At our hospital the overnight shift went from 7pm to 7am. The woman had arrived just after 5 that evening. I'd examined her at a little after 9pm. As I went through more cases, I thought back to the Asian woman. A four-hour wait isn't unheard of, but it's quite awhile to lie on a cart with the kind of pain one suffers with a broken hip. I realized they'd probably been given lower priority because the language barrier would have kept her from adequately describing the intense suffering she was enduring.

It was after 11pm when I got her x-ray. I'd had it right: a typical intertrochanteric fracture of the left hip. She would need a hip replacement.

When I returned to her I was astounded to find her still on the cart, dressed, expressionless. Nothing I'd ordered had been done! When I found her nurse I learned that she'd received her x-rays, then refused all further care.

"Who refused?" I asked. "They can't speak English."

The nurse nodded to the husband. He bowed his head, offering me a cell phone.

I took it. "Hello?" I said. "This is Dr. Kessler. Who is this?"

The woman's voice on the other end was heavily accented, but perfectly understandable. "We thank you for all you have done," she said. "Most of all we want her to be relieved of pain. Could you prescribe medicine for that, then, please, send her home?"

"I don't understand," I said, not believing my own ears.

She repeated her request.

"But she has a broken hip," I said. "She can't even stand up. This is a very serious matter, and needs immediate attention. She needs hip surgery."

"Thank you so much for your concern," said the woman, "but I must respectfully ask that you send her home."

"Uh, I will do what I can," I said, then I handed the phone back to the patient's husband. I told the nurse to call the ED administrator for an assessment. I still had patients coming in the door; they needed my attention.

At a little after 1am our overnight administrator asked me to join her with the patient and family. A third family member had arrived. This was the woman I'd spoken to on the phone. As I had suspected, she was their daughter.

I told the young woman how serious a hip fracture was. Though I was tactful and polite, I didn't spare her some of the gory details. I needed her and her parents to understand how necessary this operation was. "If she's ever going to walk again she'll need the surgery," I said.

"That's all right," said the daughter. "We thank you for your efforts. You have been most helpful. Now, if you please, we will care for her at home. She does not want the operation."

"But, ma'am, this is something we can fix," I said. "We can stop her pain, and soon she'll be walking again."

"No, thank you. She would like to be at home."

"But with the surgery she has a chance to go home to a much more normal life. Without it there are sure to be complications." I began going through it all again: "She won't be able to get up, so over time she'll probably get bedsores. With constant inactivity blood clots might develop. Often such patients get pneumonia. Does she want that?"

"If you please, she would like to go home." Though her tone was respectful almost to the point of timidity, it barely disguised the iron at her core. It was there in both women. The mother was absolutely determined to leave, and her daughter was just as determined to help her do it.

"I'm not sure what I can say to make this crystal clear," I told her. "Your mother can be saved. Except for her hip, she's in reasonably good health. If you just let us fix her hip, she has a very good chance of returning to a normal life. Yet she wants to go home, and most likely that will lead to her death, sooner rather than later... probably much sooner."

"This is what she wants," said the daughter. "This is what we want for her. She will be in the best hands with her family."

I couldn't win. Though all my training and experience told me that this case could have a good outcome, they didn't seem to think that mattered. I felt totally outgunned.

"We have a family doctor, and he might be able to help you," said the daughter.

I gave a sigh of relief. Now we were getting somewhere. She told me his name was Dr. Chu. I knew him, and felt sure he could help. Chu was a conscientious man, and, I had little doubt he would know the right way to explain all this to them. The middle-of-the-night call went out, and an hour later I was on the phone with him. I explained the injury, the family's resistance to proper treatment, and I was in the midst of my pitch for the hip replacement when he interrupted me.

"Larry", he said, " let it go. I've been their doctor for a while. They know what they want and can't be dissuaded. Have them sign an AMA[*] form, and, I'll call on them tomorrow."

"Are you serious?" I asked.

"Perfectly serious," he said. "In the end that's what will happen anyway. If you fight them all you'll be doing is delaying her from going home, and that's what she's going to do whether you and I like it or not. If she doesn't want the surgery, there's no way that they'll give in. I know them, and I'm absolutely sure that's what will happen."

I hung up, got the forms, and signed them out. I felt stymied and perplexed as the family helped the patient into a wheelchair. Despite the painkillers in her system, the move must've been excruciating; she did it with barely a grimace. The husband smiled, bowed his head again, and they were gone.

Weeks later, when I saw Dr. Chu, I asked what had happened with the woman.

"She lived for a little less than two weeks," he said. "I made three visits, but in the end she died of pneumonia."

"But how could they let that happen?" I asked. "She could've—"

---

[*] AMA: Against Medical Advice

He held up a hand, stopping me. "Larry, it's just their way."

***

In past generations many Americans from European cultures assumed that Asian people didn't put as great a value on human life as we did. The notion was as wrong then as it is now, but people from Asia, and from other cultures do have different attitudes about pain, dying and death. When an elderly person develops a life-threatening condition, such as a broken hip, they are not so quick to reverse natural processes. What we regard as standard procedure might be a "heroic measure"** to them.

Naturally, I favored the surgery. As I'd said to the daughter, the woman's overall health seemed reasonably good for her age. I didn't see anything in the break that made it more threatening than most hip fractures. With surgery she could've been going home within a short time, then, after several months of therapy, she would have every chance for a solid recovery, and however many years she had left.

But I also know that the key would be cooperation. A patient has to want to do what's necessary, and that's a lot. She would have to endure inactivity, then withstand rigorous therapy. A patient returning from a hip fracture must alter some habits, do the proper exercises, and be dependent on others to help her through the crisis. These others need to be ready and willing to do their parts. If all the right elements aren't in place, recovery becomes much more difficult. Add a cultural outlook that discourages certain methods of

---

** *heroic measure:* a treatment, procedure, or process used to avoid death. It is usually a measure that stops an immediate threat, but causes damage that would be considered unacceptable if the patient were expected to recover.

extending life, and chances of her living another six months sink dramatically.

I didn't understand exactly why this family did what they did, and I wouldn't have applied their beliefs to my own health, or that of my family. But I respect their actions. In their view, this was the way to approach death. It isn't modern medicine's place to interfere.

This was how one family dealt with a crisis of old age, injury and death. Families more grounded in western values see these things in a different way. This can be either positive or negative, as will become clear in these next two stories.

Not In My House

Not long ago the family of an Italian-American man brought him into our ER. The man's illness was obvious. His appearance had deteriorated to the point where any guess at his age would have been futile, but his records showed that he was in his late-60s. His emaciated body was jaundiced to the point of turning bronze. His hair had thinned, and his arms and legs were like sticks. In the midst of all this was an abdomen, bursting with fluid. His belly button had popped up like the timer on a Thanksgiving turkey. Cherry angiomata (red spots that are the hallmark of liver disease) speckled his torso. His disease was pancreatic cancer. He was terminal.

A small, timid woman stayed by his side. I soon learned this was his wife. She and her husband had been accompanied to the ER by two young men and their wives. The men were the couples' sons.

Though the father looked terrible, his family appeared to be prosperous. When I spoke to the son the conversation quickly shifted from his father's care to cars. He sold them, and asked what I drove. When I told him he advised me it was time to move up. "You're the kind of guy who would have a great time with a Porsche," he said. "You'd appreciate everything about it."

When an affluent family brings someone into the ER it's usually because of an accident, injury, or a sudden change for the worse in an already ill patient. At first I assumed this was an example of the last option, but I soon realized there was more to it than that.

When I looked at the patient's list of medications, I said to the son: "You know your father is terminal, don't you?"

"Of course we do," said the son. "He was diagnosed with pancreatic cancer months ago. Not long after that they told us he wouldn't get better."

"I'm not sure I understand," I said. "He's in very bad shape. Has anyone approached you about terminal care, and end-of-life decisions?"

"Sure," said the son. "We had hospice care, but it just wasn't working."

"What was wrong?"

"The old man wants to die at home in his bed. I can't blame him, but it's just not how things work anymore. Right, doc?"

"People do it," I said. "That's what hospice care was designed for. You must've received some counseling about that."

"Yeah, but the whole thing was really a pipedream," said the son. "You know... he's got this idea that he'll just lie there, and close his eyes, and die nice and peaceful, going to his reward, and all that. But that's not how it happens. It's all tubes and tanks, and shit and piss, and a stench you wouldn't believe."

"I just can't have that in my house," said the man's wife. As she approached us she glanced over at the stretcher where the patient lay. The patient's wife never left his side.

"We just want him to die peacefully," said the son, "and believe me, with him lying there at home, there's no peace at all."

"You can't provide your dad with a healthy environment?"

"It's not unhealthy. It's just... well... he disrupts things."

"I'm not sure I understand," I said. "Does he try to cause physical disturbances?"

"Of course not," said the daughter-in-law. "He can't even get out of bed. But just the fact that he's there, dying—well, it's taken over the whole house. He's not just an old man who's sick in his room. He soils the sheets, needs this, that, or the other, and I just can't take all those smells. I can't do this—not in my house."

I looked down at the father's recent medical data. "You have a nurse there round the clock."

"The nurses do help," said the son.

"But still, there's just so much to do," said his wife. "I was never trained to clean up after someone like..." She broke off, staring across at her in-laws.

After his wife went over to the admissions desk to answer questions, the son said: "She was never too wild about this hospice stuff. Don't get me wrong. We were ready to go along with it to make Dad feel better. He's my dad. We woulda done anything to make him feel better. But the truth is, he's never gonna feel better again. It's all downhill from here, and my wife just can't take it. She's sensitive... always has been."

"But hospice care is meant to help families care for their loved ones in the home, so that patients can die peacefully, with their families there, and without hospitalization," I said.

The son shrugged. "Yeah, I know that's the idea, but sometimes it just doesn't work. We had him on chemo, but a few weeks ago he stopped. He said he didn't want to do it anymore—no expensive treatments, no big surgeries—just let the cancer do its stuff. He thought he'd be gone in a couple of weeks, and we did too. So we started with the hospice people. They made it all sound peaceful, just like I said before—like he was just gonna close his eyes, and that would be that. But it didn't happen."

That didn't make sense to me. Hospice workers are trained to help families and patients face the realities of death. "What triggered your bringing him in tonight?" I asked.

"Uh..." The son had to think for a moment. "He's been hurting... I mean, really bad. I guess the painkillers aren't doing it anymore. Anyway, it wasn't really any one thing... just that he's hurting so bad, and all that stuff my wife was talking about."

I glanced over at his wife. She stood by the desk, filling out a form, while muttering to no one in particular: "I just can't have it in my house. We're not ready. Nobody's ready..."

The hospitalist who'd admitted the patient approached me, and we went behind a door for privacy. "There's not much we can do," he said. "He might go anytime. He knows that. He says he wants to die at home."

"But his family brought him in here," I said. "They don't seem prepared to take him."

"What's wrong? Didn't the hospice caregivers give them counseling?"

"I would think they did all they could, but you know as well as I do, some people can't deal with it, no matter how much coaching they get. It looks like that's what we have here."

As the doctor and I talked, we were still within sight of the patient and his wife. I thought about talking to the patient's wife, but when I met the elderly woman's eyes she immediately glanced away. She turned her attention back to her husband, gently tucking in a blanket. She wanted him to be comfortable, and had no clue how to do it. I could see that this couple was beyond making choices. They'd lived their lives, raised their children, and now they could do no more. This decision would fall on the next generation.

The sons went along with their wives. There was no longer a place at home for this sick old man. He would be "better off" there at the hospital, they said. How could I dispute them? If they weren't willing to do what was necessary to allow him to die at home, all the counseling on earth couldn't change that. If we were to turn him away there could be repercussions, both legal and extra legal. Desperate family members had been known to euthanize their terminal relatives, often botching the job, inflicting pain, and getting caught. Also there have been cases where hospitals and healthcare professionals have been sued successfully for refusing care. In today's medical environment we must always consider the legal side.

The hospital did what it felt it had to do. We admitted him. We eased his pain, administering a high dose of narcotics right there at the Emergency Dock. These painkillers acted quickly, allowing the patient to sleep. His sleep was terminal. He died there in the hospital two days later. With his family by his side, his head lay on a pillow he'd brought from home. The family returned to a home free of dirty sheets, bedpans, and tubes. They felt it was better that way.

***

One of the problems in our own culture is that it doesn't provide us with the emotional tools to accept death. Dying is no easier than living. Like the son in this story noted, it's not just lying back peacefully, and taking one's last breath. It's a process with ups and downs, and after a certain point, it always ends the same way. We all die once.

The conveniences of modern life are designed to insulate us from nature. We live in newly-built or refurbished homes with all the modern-day comforts. Drainpipes, sewers, and sanitation systems take away all our excesses with barely any effort from us. Using these tools, we can usually keep life's physical messes contained. We solve most physically offensive problems with a flush of the toilet or a trip to the garbage can. This is such a basic part of our standard of living that many of us see it as the minimum that we can accept in cleanliness and comfort.

At the same time we have traditions, emotions, and, sometimes, financial considerations, that often make dying at home the best alternative. That's what's fueled the growth of hospice care in the last few decades. Hospice staffers are trained to help patients and their families deal with the physical and emotional hardships of death. Hospice workers have successfully helped millions through the processes of death, grieving and acceptance, but when family members simply aren't willing, there's little anyone can do.

This was a family that could not deal with the final stages of dying. To them home was a haven from discomfort, inconvenience and mess. Death had no place there. Death was a tragic event best relegated to an institutional setting. A hospital staff deals with death every day, so isn't that where it should happen? That seemed to be this family's attitude.

If we could've somehow persuaded them to take their father home, it's likely that he would've suffered more physical pain than he did with us. At home he would've been receiving the same pain medication, but in a home setting there's often fear of giving the dosages necessary to deal with the pain associated with the end of life. No family member wants the responsibility or onus of "losing" this patient. We worry that we will see ourselves as murderers. Most of us fear the possibility of taking of another's life as much as we fear death itself. In that sense, moving him from his home to the hospital may have been the right choice. In an atmosphere that can't accept death, dying gets far more complicated, and often that makes it more painful.

Choice

It was a rare thing to see in the ED: a slow afternoon. This seldom happened on Friday, when understaffed nursing homes often sent their overflow to the hospital for the weekend. If the patient didn't have visitors scheduled at the nursing home, and their already short staff was down to bare bones, then the home would select that patient as one of the ones who needed some extra care that weekend. It was easy to make a case for it. These were the old and the sick. We could always find a reason to admit them for a couple of days, and the red tape involved in saying no created an inducement to simply let them in.

But on this particular Friday we seemed to have a reprieve from our most plentiful weekend guests. In addition to the dearth of nursing home extras, we had far fewer young gunshot victims than we normally saw, and all the other usual traumas were under control. Some of us were actually talking about plans for a leisurely weekend.

That's when I heard the voice on the radio override the static: "Unit 2, Unit 2, ALS in route with elderly male, cardiac arrest, ETA: five minutes."

Once we knew a cardiac arrest case was coming, we began preparations immediately. When an elderly male's heart stops, he has a poor prognosis from the start. It's a situation that brought one of my earliest mentors to comment: "Came in dead, stayed that way." Still, though death resists all attempts at reversal, it's our job to try.

In this case our efforts were almost stopped in their tracks by the overzealous medics. Pushing a loaded gurney, they burst through the emergency doors, then careened around the first corner like pit mechanics rolling a car back onto the track at Indianapolis Speedway. One corner of the stretcher sideswiped a wall, slowing them down. Suddenly the medics remembered their cargo, and straightened up.

As the staff descended on the body, I asked the usual questions about who this was, when it happened, and what had already been done. The young medic in the lead told me of his on-site assessment and treatment of the patient: asystole (no heartbeat), which he'd treated with three rounds of epinephrine, atropine and CPR. The patient made no response to these efforts. I assessed the patient's rhythm, confirmed his asystole condition, and told my team to stop. It was no longer sensible to try to resuscitate this man. Even if we could get a heartbeat going, it would only pump blood through an otherwise lifeless body. You can't give life support when there's no life to begin with. I concluded my order by stating the time. The clock on the wall said: 3:29pm.

As the excitement ended, I looked to the medic and asked: "Where's his family?"

"The PD has the wife behind us," he said, meaning that the police were bringing her, and she would be there momentarily.

I gathered the paperwork on the case, and as I sat at a desk, writing, a nurse came in and told me: "The arrest patient's wife is here."

Now came the part every doctor hates: having to tell a family member that a loved one is dead. This is when old age, grievous injury, and even the ravages of disease mean nothing. Though the patient may have endured years of incredible pain, or long months in a coma, the end must always be explained. The living must be consoled with the idea that no effort was spared in preserving some spark of life in the patient's body. It's always a variation on the we-tried-everything talk. It's not false because, in fact, we do try everything and then some. That's what modern medicine trains us to do.

Every doctor has his own version, altering it to fit individual circumstances. Some doctors tell families their loved ones have "passed away" or "gone on." I'm not comfortable with such language. Other doctors prefer the word "expired," perhaps because it sounds both official and neutral. I don't like that one at all. Milk expires, people die.

When we need to state the facts of death officially, we write it down. If we need to be emotionally neutral to keep ourselves functioning, we do that only in the privacy of our own thoughts. For the patient and his or her family we should have the respect to admit that death has occurred, and to tell them why. We should do it in a sensitive way that avoids both brutality and artificial closeness. In that spirit, I also stay away from the standard, "I'm sorry." This is supposed to be an explanation, not an apology. Behind it should be a sense of empathy, but your primary role here is to help the family get an immediate sense of what just happened. This requires honesty. It doesn't mean you have to describe every grimy detail of death, but for me it does mean that I avoid phrases like: "The patient didn't suffer any pain." I don't know how dying feels, so I don't try to talk about something of which I know nothing.

In this instance I was preparing to have this talk with the patient's 80-year-old wife. I first saw her sitting outside the patient's room. She still had her winter coat on. Obviously in the habit of always looking her best, she appeared to have just had her silver hair tinted to perfection. This was one of those remarkable women who can be 80, look 80, and make 80 look like a great age. To use an old saying that works despite inflation: she looked like a million bucks.

She sat, listening quietly, as I introduced myself, and told her what had happened to her husband. She smiled at me, thanked me politely and asked: "Can I see him?"

"Of course," I said, "in just a few moments, as soon as the nurses prepare the room." That meant they were still cleaning up the blood, getting rid of the needles, and dealing with the physical disarray that often accompanies an attempt at resuscitation. As I stood up I saw my nurse giving me the signal that all was ready.

I walked the woman to the threshold of her husband's room. She stood at the door forever, and I wondered if she was going to collapse. I was about to offer to help her into a chair, but before I could she was moving to his bedside. She took his hand, bent over and kissed his forehead. "Thank you for fifty-five wonderful years," she said softly. "I'll be with you soon, my love" As she stood I realized that her eyes were dry. Her tiny face wore a glorious smile as she straightened up, and walked out of the room. It was the rest of us who were crying.

Many times since I've remembered that woman. When her beloved husband died she chose a celebration of their lives over mourning. She made this amazing decision quickly, simply, and without the guidance of anyone there. Her courage was in allowing herself to see this choice was possible. It honored him, it honored her, and it recognized all that they'd had together. What more can one ask?

***

Though all three of these stories involve families, doctors, and the process of death, the attitudes about death on display here couldn't be more different. In the first story people from an eastern culture accepted pain, disruption, grief, and death itself, all within their home. The woman had suffered the break, but not knowing its severity, she came in for a diagnosis. Had it been something less serious, where she could've begun her recovery and gone home in a day or two, they probably would have been fine with that. But this was something more difficult. Recovery would require cooperation from her and her family. If she was going to be alive in 6 months she would have a lot of hard work to do-starting now. The same would be true of her family. Her background, attitude, and temperament allowed her to choose a different course. It wasn't what I would've done, but the longer I thought about it, the more I came to respect her choice. She did what she felt was right, and her family fully supported her.

The second family was a product of our own culture. Though their hospice staff could provide many services, in the end nothing could change the family's ingrained attitudes. The only way they might've avoided this last ditch trip to the hospital would've been if their father had died quickly, at home. That would've spared them the mess, and made them feel good about keeping him there. But it didn't happen that way. When he lingered it tested their abilities, and in the end they couldn't endure it. Like many of us, they'd been acclimated to distancing themselves from death, and all that went with it. They could sit by his bed as he died, but only if that bed was in a hospital room, at a far remove from their spotless home.

The third story might offer a clue to something better. Here was another elderly person dying. In his case, he was already gone when he reached us. He'd lived a long life, but, as is true of every one of us, at the end his body broke down. His heart stopped. He died. His wife, who was only a little younger, followed him to the hospital, visited with the body of the man she'd loved, and honored his memory. As she looked at him for the last time, her smile was one of bravery, memory, and celebration. If only we could all deal with death so well. We should try. We all die once.

Chapter Two: Preservation

We are taught to preserve life. This isn't only true of doctors. Our parents, teachers, coaches, counselors, and every other source of conventional wisdom and authority, have drummed the same idea into all of us: If there is life there's hope, so any life-saving measure is justified.

In particular circumstances, when faced with the issue of survival, whether hypothetical or real, we might temporarily suspend this practice. If grandma lies in her last coma, and the processes of life threaten to strip her of all dignity, we might decide it's time to pull the plug. This decision is almost always preceded by consultation with doctors, relatives, and spiritual advisors. Sometimes the decision takes hours, while some families puzzle over it for weeks and months. For others it isn't a decision at all; it's simply one more instance where life must continue, no matter what the cost.

If there is a default setting in the emergency room, it's this one. We're in the business of saving lives. We do it without the benefit of careful consideration of future consequences. It's not that all medical professionals think that every sign of life must be supported without regard to outcome. The problem is time. A human being comes in the door with a life-threatening illness or injury, and our first priority is to bring whatever life is there to a stable, sustainable condition as quickly as possible. If we fail, the patient dies. If we succeed, the rest of the medical profession takes over.

When all we see is evidence of the patient's catastrophe, yet clear signs of life—or even its possibility—are present, we try to save the patient. The urge to save a life can often cloud our judgment. It seems like such a good goal, but in the field of emergency medicine one good goal can easily collide with another.

Saving a life is a sensible goal as long as the life is worth living. What makes life worthwhile? Each of us has a different answer. An athletic outdoorsman might find the loss of his legs cuts all the worthwhile life out from under him. At the same time, someone who already lives with a permanent disability is far more likely to appreciate the possibilities of spending the rest of her life in a wheelchair.

But sometimes the view is quite clear. When we step back from a case, and look at all that went into it, we might get a better sense of the pitfalls and possibilities arriving in ERs every day.

Amazement

They tell us that residency training prepares a young doctor for anything—almost. The "almost" crashed through the trauma bay's sliding doors at 3am.

It was a typical night in the neighborhood, which meant we were dealing with crises nonstop. I was the ER's senior resident. I attended to some cases myself, while assigning others to the junior residents. I'd long since become accustomed to making decisions amidst chaos, and this night, like almost all others, had required that skill. As I directed this case here, and that one over there, I began to feel like a traffic cop.

Suddenly we heard a crash, and the sound of glass shattering. Our latest patient had arrived without the benefit of ambulance, or any other medical escort. The non-medical escorts he did have weren't waiting around to see how he made out. They'd hurled him from their car without even coming to a full stop. The sliding doors' smashed glass was like a calling card. We all knew what this one would be: a victim of gang violence.

It was a familiar scenario in that part of Queens. Our trauma bay's sliding doors opened onto a street scene where strip clubs and bakeries thrived side-by-side. There were people living there who worked, and struggled to keep their kids on the straight-and-narrow. There were alcoholics and addicts too far gone to care. And there were the gangs. The gangs were like a subterranean society, just barely visible by day, but permeating the whole atmosphere at night. They were the cause of peoples' grilled windows and the sliding metal mesh that covered every storefront at closing time. The gangs were what spurred local schools to beef up their security. Parents fought them, feared them, and denied their existence, but the gangs lived on. And here, lying in a spray of shattered glass, was one of their victims. Was this kid a member? An initiate? A civilian caught in crossfire? Were drugs involved? Or could it be a grudge killing? We would never know, but the idea that this patient's arrival and condition might be anything other than gang-related seemed somewhere between ludicrous and impossible.

We scooped up the victim as gently as possible, and placed him on the trauma cart. I glanced around and saw everyone taking out trauma shears: enlarged scissors, with colorful handles, and a bottom blade flattened at the end to avoid punctures. The blades are strong enough and sharp enough to cut through a penny. Trauma shears can cut the clothes from a victim in seconds, revealing the true scope of the emergency team's job.

We stripped the patient, and the nurses brought in a cervical collar to protect his neck against effects from a possible injury there. One of the interns was searching the patient's arms for likely veins for an IV. The second-year residents started checking ABCs: airway, breathing, and circulation. This was all standard procedure.

I stood on a footstool, directing the scene as if it were a complex shot in a movie. One resident called out: "Several entry wounds in chest." The anesthesia resident was trying to intubate the patient when she suddenly realized her gloves were dripping with blood. It came from a head wound. "His right pupil is fixed and dilated," she announced. The cardiac monitor began by displaying chaotic heart rhythm, which means little. These rhythms were simply evidence that there was electrical activity; there was no pulse. I ordered one resident to do a bedside ultrasound of the heart. That would show if there was any cardiac activity. There wasn't. Still, this had been a young healthy male until he met with a bullet. My first instinct as a doctor, and as a human being, was to make him well.

Once we had him intubated, on a ventilator, with IVs pouring fresh blood and fluids into him, the next step would be CPR. For this we had to decide whether to crack open his chest and perform open cardiac massage.

That's when my attending physician, Dr. Sachter came in. "What have we got?" he asked.

I drew a breath, went through the steps in my head, and quickly gave him the necessary data. He looked from me to the patient. At that moment all of us had our eyes on the body, and finally it sank in. This victim was just a kid. He was big enough that he might've been mistaken for a fully-grown young man, but now it was clear that he couldn't be more than 13 or 14.

"We should open him up," I said. "He's young. He's strong. He might make it."

Dr. Sachter shook his head. "No. He's gone." He then mentioned several persuasive statistics on postmortem thoracotomies. He was right, and I knew it. I'd just needed enough time to process what was in front of me. This boy had been shot dead, and there was nothing I could do about it.

From behind us we heard a metallic clink as something hit the tile floor. We looked around to see one of the techs picking up the boy's clothes. Several small cylinders rolled across the tile, stopping within a foot or two of the body. They were nine millimeter bullets spilling out from the victim's own pocket. The sight of them left us sad, but not surprised.

That's when the screams caught up with the body. We heard the woman's shrieks for several seconds before she burst into the trauma bay, security close on her heels. This large, shaking woman looked down at her son, and was stunned into silence.

Dr. Sachter, leaned toward me, and whispered: "Pronounce the time of death." He started toward the dazed mother, ready to calm her.

At that moment the mother screamed: "Oh, God, take me now, Jesus, take me now! How? How?" For a moment it was as if she'd swallowed her words, then she cried softly: "He'd just gone to the library. That's all. How can this be?"

No one could give her an answer.

The woman's screams rose up again, and some of our people accompanied her from the trauma bay. She followed the cart carrying her son's lifeless body. I heard the paradoxical sound of louder and louder screams fading into the distance. Their echoes rang through my head.

As I gazed at the bullets, I realized she'd never known anything about them. Her son had either been with a gang, or he lived in mortal fear of them—perhaps both—yet he'd managed to keep it hidden. I wondered how a mother and son living in the same house could lead such separate lives. She lived in a home where her son did his homework, and sometimes visited the library. He lived in a violent world where guns, bullets, and blood were normal commodities. He'd let his mom think that his daily routine was mostly one of study. Did he worry that she would learn his secret? Somewhere deep down did she know? I thought of how we all hide things from each other, some small, some large. Much of modern medicine depends on this deception.

Modern medicine can keep almost any body alive. I wanted to save the young boy because it seemed possible. Despite the massive head wound and the stopped heart, we could have brought life back into this body. Did I think of the quality of that life? Did I consider the body that would lie in a bed, or slump in a wheelchair? Did I take into account the sadness of a strong young boy reduced to nothing more than stale breaths and regulated heartbeats? I didn't have the time or training for those thoughts. The only place where they could originate was in the area of common sense. Like the young victim's mother, I closed my eyes to things that were right in front of me—practically a necessity in medicine today.

Survival by Coincidence

One morning, not far from the hospital in Queens, a 35-year-old woman we'll call "Gloria" was walking to work. As Gloria was turning a corner a man with a gun was pulling a holdup. His victim had just handed over the cash when suddenly something went wrong. Was it a car backfire? Or the sight of a cop? Or a witness shouting? No one really knew, but the robber's gun went off. The bullet traveled about a hundred feet, then punctured Gloria's chest and went out her back. In that first instant she literally didn't know what hit her.

She figured it out in the moment after she'd fallen. She'd been shot, and had no idea how or why. She was conscious, and when the ambulance got her to our trauma bay she was still aware. She was even talking.

Though Gloria's life was quickly fading, none of us knew that yet. She'd been shot in the chest, but it seemed the bullet had passed completely through, exiting her back. We weren't even sure if any vital organs were damaged. However, we quickly realized the bullet must have come close to her heart. It even might've nicked it.

Gloria arrived at exactly the right moment. Earlier that morning a patient had arrived in the ER with an aneurysm. It was one of those rare cases where we could get the hospital's elite specialists, the cardiothoracic surgeons, down to our dock. These are the ones who do bypasses. These are the hands that transplant hearts. These are the folks who make the impossible possible. They're good, they know it, and their time is valuable. They don't leave their upstairs quarters for just any old case. In Queens an arriving gunshot victim, still talking, wouldn't be something they would run downstairs to see. A visit from these guys meant an obvious threat to life, and a clear solution that absolutely required their presence; it took an aneurysm.

When Gloria came in the cardiothoracic surgeons had wrapped up their work, and were about to go back upstairs where they could save lives at a more sane and leisurely pace. But then they saw this crazy gunshot wound. We'd located the entry and exit wounds, and were still in the process of resuscitation. We were following our standard procedures.

Then the cardiothoracic team took over. This was when Gloria's case turned into the kind of miracle you only see in TV hospital dramas. They examined the damage, assessed the situation in seconds, then got her into an elevator, and up to an operating room. When they opened her they found something no one had expected. On its way through her body the bullet had pierced her heart. This shot-in-a-million had gone into her chest, punctured a hole in her atria, then exited her back. Had it hit the larger aorta she would've been dead. These pros knew what to do. In a lengthy operation they stopped the internal bleeding, and repaired the damage well enough that her heart could begin functioning again. They saved Gloria's life, and put her on the road to recovery.

It was a miracle: a timely presence and split-second decisions combining to stop a death. This combination gave decades of worthwhile life to a victim of random violence. It was good, right, and just in the best traditions of medicine.

It was also an accident.

Save My Dad

Guns punch holes in people of all ages, with outcomes ranging from the mundane to the tragic and on to the miraculous. When a bullet doesn't immediately kill its victim, it often leaves us with life-and-death decisions. Many of these choices arrive suddenly and inevitably. On occasion we get it wrong. Whenever that happens, we like to think that, given more time, we would have done better.

But take the son who came out one morning to get the morning paper, only to find his elderly father lying there, victim of a fall. Even before his fall, the old man had been failing. Dementia had sapped his mind, and age had worn down his body. His life was drawing to a close.

He lay at the bottom of the steps, fully clothed. He might have been a homeless person sleeping. When the son tried to rouse him, the father didn't respond. When the father arrived as a patient at our dock, our first thoughts were stroke, or diabetic coma.

It wasn't either one. Quickly we found evidence of his fall in the form of a broken neck and hip. This poor fellow's time had come.

As I began to brief the son on his father's condition, he began to tremble. "He's my dad," he said. "You've got to save him."

"We'll do everything we can for him," I said, "but if he does survive you should understand what his life will be like." I began to describe the most essential details in the life of a human vegetable: bed sores, infections, pneumonia, and all the rest. I didn't get far.

"Save him," he reiterated. "I don't care what it takes, you've got to save my dad."

Why did the son want to save him? No one can ever be sure about someone else's thought processes, but we can all sympathize with a child wanting to save a father. Guilt may have played a role. When children or old people fall victim to their own actions, we often find ways to blame ourselves. Had the door to the steps been left open? How long had it been since anyone had checked on this old fellow? When we go searching for reasons, what we find can be disturbing. Once we feel the pain of guilt, we'll do almost anything to make it go away. The most obvious way for this distraught son to do that was to try to save his dad—or at least get us to do it.

There were things we could do. We could stabilize his father, and even begin some healing processes, but none of these would be of any real consequence. We could keep him "comfortable," whatever that meant. This was one of those cases where "comfortable" simply meant we didn't see any signs that he was in pain. It was doubtful that he would regain even the diminished mental capacity he'd had before his injuries. He was well on the way to becoming the thing no one wants to be: the classic "vegetable."

We did what we could in the ER, then the rest of the medical system took him. The hope was that he could improve enough to be transferred to a convalescent facility. Theoretically he'd be going there to heal. But before he could do that he would have to show some hopeful signs of life. This old guy simply didn't have that capacity. Though he survived several surgeries, each was just a stopgap measure fixing some specific difficulty. His was a body too far gone to care. Each operation saved him for another. Each problem punctuated the truth: he would never go anywhere again.

He died three months later.

The Will to Die

We've all seen moments when the body and mind work together. The most obvious examples are in sports, where these tandem efforts are often as beautiful as they are spectacular. Watch an Olympic gymnast working through a routine, or a sprinter crossing the finish line of a 100-meter race. These are the celebrated moments when mind meets body creating a flow of thought, energy and muscle.

These cooperative efforts don't stop on the field. Though they may not be so obvious or celebrated, the links between the mind and body are always there, from a baby's cry to a death rattle. As a body ages and deteriorates, and the brain perceives this loss, the conscious and unconscious often decide that the body's time has come. In times gone by that was when the patient succumbed. In those days, what most people hoped for in their final moments was peace.

Today, when we have more control of dying than we've ever had, peace is often a casualty on the road to death.

On a winter day about two years ago we received a homeless man who appeared to be dead. In medicine we give death some hoops to jump through before we'll admit it's really there. We have good reasons for most of these, including the requirement that under certain conditions a cooling body lacking measurable vital signs, still can't be declared dead until it's "warm and dead." In other words, we have to reheat the body to learn whether it's a corpse or a patient. Only a temperature near normal can tell us for sure. That's what we did with this homeless man.

The homeless man had gone into cardiac arrest. When the emergency responders brought him in, he had no breath, no pulse, and his temperature was 89° Fahrenheit. This was a case where going by the book meant rewarming the body. In rewarming there are two options: passive, which means warm air, blankets, and other external applications, and active, which entails more complex methods of internal rewarming through intubation and irrigation of the stomach and bladder with warm saline fluids.

The man was roughly 60 years old. In his current condition he looked very dead. In our rush to revive him, we couldn't do a full examination, but I imagined he'd been in poor health before his heart stopped. Nonetheless, we intubated him, and began the active warming process. Around 94° we got a heartbeat. He was going to live, for the moment.

We had no records on him, so we scanned him and gave him a chest X-ray. What we saw didn't reflect robust health, but there were no broken bones. The chest x-ray showed indications of illness. A week later they found him in the records of an upstate hospital. He had metastatic liver cancer. It had spread.

This wasn't a patient who would ever wake up. If he'd known the options, it's doubtful he would've wanted to. If, by some miracle, we'd been able to bring him back to consciousness, his world would've been one of pain. To relieve the pain he would've needed powerful suppressants and sedatives. This would've gone on until he either slipped back into a coma, or died. But he was already in a coma, and if his body had been able to do what it was meant to do, it would have died then-and-there. It didn't. Medical science intervened.

Once he left us he went to the Intensive Care Unit, or ICU. For many of us this is where the last, most expensive days of our lives are lived. Some of us are luckier. Some of us die at home. Some of us die at the scenes of accidents or crimes, and some of us die on the way to the hospital. Some of us die in the other hospital wards, when a sudden crisis overtakes us and kills us almost immediately. But if we survive the ambulance ride, or burst blood vessel, or the emergency surgery, then we go to the ICU. Some of us are lucky enough to leave there, and recover. Some are transferred to less intensive, less expensive care (though many of these return to the ICU). But for many terminal patients Intensive Care is the last, and sometimes longest, stop of their lives. That's where our homeless man went.

That's where his upstate records went. And that is where the efforts to prolong his life went.

By the time his records arrived the team in ICU already knew most of what was there. They could see the cancer. It had entered his lungs, which was one reason his chest x-ray had looked far from perfect. Having consumed most of his liver, it was now traveling far and wide. One-by-one his organs began to fail. Lungs, stomach and kidneys were all barely functioning. Though they managed to keep his heart beating, there was little or no brain function. He remained comatose. His kidneys failed, so they put him on dialysis. Still, his heart kept going.

Dialysis is the process of cleaning the blood. That's what a kidney does. It's difficult, labor-intensive, and hugely expensive. At its best it keeps a patient alive, and functioning pretty well, until a better alternative emerges, such as a transplant. Even when dialysis patients can't be cured, often the treatment gives them a chance to function in everyday life. But dialysis can become a bizarre treatment prolonging life that's human in name only. That's what happened here.

We had a body where nature was completing its cycle. We cheated nature and we cheated death. Worst of all we cheated the patient. Nature had no closure, death had no corpse, and the patient was stripped of any dignity he might've had. He'd almost died homeless in the streets, very possibly after a sad life. Instead he was brought to us. We might've simply made sure he suffered no discomfort, and allowed him to die in peace. Peace was what his body was aiming for, but we wouldn't give it to him. His final struggle was an effort to die. We wouldn't let him.

In dialysis his blood pressure dropped steadily. Finally his other organs failed. About two weeks later the homeless man died with no one to mourn his passing. If there'd been any mourning it shouldn't have been for his death; all grief should have been directed at the way he'd passed. That was our handiwork.

***

In today's hospital we can keep some bodies alive almost indefinitely. Even the 13-year-old gunshot victim might've lived for some time if we'd known about his imminent arrival. If we'd been prepared for his wounds, we could've made his heart beat again, but we couldn't have brought him back to consciousness. Though religious authorities might debate whether his soul was still there, we might've kept the door open to a minimally functioning body. Oxygen would enter and escape his lungs. The heart would beat, and the other organs below the brain would function. Though we often give lip service to the idea that life is fragile, as long as modern medicine is standing by, it's not that easy to kill someone. Look at Gloria, the other gunshot victim. She came in with a hole through her heart, and left us healing.

Modern medicine gives us miracles, but in doing so it also presents us with choices. Should we always want these miracles? Is saving a life so that a body can be a vegetable a miracle? Or a magic trick? When the only goal of medicine is keeping a near-corpse alive, the people in charge should ask these questions.

Chapter Three: At What Cost?

People don't become doctors because they aspire to produce human vegetables. Most of us start out with the dream of curing people. This doesn't mean doctors are more altruistic than anyone else. By the time you're an undergrad selecting pre-med courses, you already realize that medicine is more complex than that. Some of those undergrads see medicine in terms of high pay. Others want the respect that goes with an ancient and absolutely necessary profession. Some fall in love with the power inherent in healing. Nevertheless, most young people recognize the core mission of medicine as helping people get well.

Our attitudes about medicine form early. They originate with our parents, and in our initial experiences with medical professionals. If we have good experiences with our pediatrician, we're more likely to see medicine in a positive light for the rest of our lives. If we distrust our first doctor, that doubt will infuse our attitudes toward healthcare throughout adulthood.

Media plays an important role in our perceptions. For my generation America's family doctor was Marcus Welby, M.D. Played by Robert Young (whose previous TV hit was an early sitcom called "Father Knows Best"), Dr. Welby was an idealized anachronism even when the show first ran in 1969. He was the small-town doctor who made house calls. He was wise, comforting, and incredibly competent. Though not all of his patients recovered, no viewer could doubt that Dr. Welby's care was the best anyone could ever hope to receive. He was assisted by a much younger physician named Dr. Kiley, but it was the older, more experienced Welby whose approach usually prevailed.

Welby had been preceded on the tube by Dr. Kildare, Ben Casey, and numerous other movie and TV physicians. Their descendants still practice on "House" and "Grey's Anatomy." Today's TV doctors are more likely to visit patients in their hospital beds than in their homes, but they live by the same rules: Each patient awaits a medical miracle. The doctors make their best efforts, and come through most of the time. When they don't there's always a clear life lesson.

In the past most medical shows and movies relied on stories of patients with life-threatening conditions. We would first see them in a hospital bed, or a doctor's office, receiving the terrible prognosis. Obstacles to recovery were endless. The patient might need some new kind of surgery that our hero has never before performed, or a drug that's still in the testing stage. Some shows dealt with people's religious or cultural qualms about medical intervention. If a patient did die, the plot might go into how the doctor helped the survivors deal with their grief. There were few ambulances, practically no emergency rooms, and dramatic high points almost always depended on the idea that the doctor should, could, and would bring about the best possible result. Any characters who doubted this were portrayed in a negative light.

Modern medical shows are grittier, and more "realistic." Surgeons get more bloodstains, and patients have more doubts. ERs aren't just common; they gave the prototype of today's medical shows its name. George Clooney played Dr. Doug Ross on *ER*, one of the biggest hits of the '90s. Dr. Ross was a fitting successor to Welby. Ross dealt with similar crises, but because he first saw most patients when they were lying on a gurney, there was a new edge to it: the immediacy of the setting. Today's shows are set where the action is. The life-threatening situations don't develop in the first act; they're clear from the first shot. Even before the ambulance siren drones down, we know this patient is in big, sudden trouble. Otherwise he or she wouldn't be here.

When the focus isn't on emergency medicine, it shifts to procedures and ethics. In the old shows most ethical conflicts were defined with painful honesty by the doctors themselves. If doctors disagreed, it was almost always about procedures. One would favor the conservative course, the other would believe in a more radical approach. If doctors disagreed with their patients, their differences usually grew from an emotional conflict, or religious qualms. Though they seldom named specific religions, those old shows seemed to have a lot of quasi-Christian Scientists whose faith barred them from accepting medical treatment. TV doctors always wound up either sadly shaking their heads, or finding a method that allowed the family to give in without compromising their beliefs. The dual lesson was always the same: we must respect the faiths of others, but if we would just do what the doctor says we would all survive and thrive.

Newer hospital dramas deal with 21st century reality: it's the doctors we don't trust. Some are incompetent, others are greedy, and all are caught up in a system that's often crazy. Yet even these new shows hold up the motivation to heal as the ruling factor in their characters' lives. The doctors who are more concerned with money, power, or status are regarded as villains, or, at the least, deeply flawed antagonists. Our heroes are still those doctors who save peoples' lives just because they're dedicated to healing.

People go to medical school for all kinds of reasons. I was prodded to do it by my father. He believed that the best professions were those where others need you more than you need them. Someone else might be fascinated by the science, or the mystery, but we all study medicine in the same cultural atmosphere. TV, movies, and novels reflect and reinforce that atmosphere. Though the newer shows might portray bad doctors, these are always balanced by good doctors who care deeply about their patients. These shows teach us what we know about medical ethics.

When an aspiring student finishes high school most of his or her understanding of modern medicine comes from family attitudes, personal observations, and the media. Our student will take pre-med courses, but in undergrad studies there won't be much about medical ideals or ethics. When our student reaches medical school the only time ethics are sure to be covered is in the issue of end-of-life care. It's centered around the idea of resuscitate-and-revive. You're taught to do all it takes to preserve life. The principles surrounding "permissive death" (a more positive way of saying "do not resuscitate") aren't even discussed.

This lopsided attitude permeates all things medical, from hit TV dramas to actual ERs. It has no place for an Asian family that wants mom to come home to die. If a story has a 13-year-old dying from gang violence, that happens at the beginning, and resolves into a lesson learned by the end. Why? Because hopelessness doesn't make for a good story.

When we carry a story's ideals into real situations, the ideals often lose. Take the 42-year-old father of two who got caught in the middle of a car chase. A cop car smashed into him, and he arrived at our dock with a C-4 neck fracture. There was little we could do but keep him alive. We did that, and when he became conscious he couldn't move or feel anything below his neck. He couldn't speak. All he could do was blink his eyes. In our workup we found his spine was severed. Our best healing efforts could give him nothing more than a lifetime in a wheelchair. Every thought he would ever express would have to come through those blinking eyes. Do our medical schools try to make ethical sense out of this? No. Their best answer is to keep him alive at all costs. The best reason they can give for this is a vague and untenable hope that somehow medicine will one day heal severed spinal cords. If there's a second-best reason it's the notion that life is better than death—no matter what.

Beyond this are the more everyday ethics concerning prevention, diagnosis, treatments, and most of all: access. Most of what concerns us about healthcare, both private and public, is access. That's at the heart of debates about rationing. It's the core concern in the development of new drugs and therapies: who gets them first? It's the first thing any of us want to know when we hear about a new procedure that affects us: Can we get it now? If we're insured well enough we might. If we're uninsured we probably won't.

We've all heard the horror stories about the uninsured. Almost any working doctor, including me, can recite dozens of them. For instance, one day about eighteen months ago a man came in with absolutely no insurance. He was noticeably overweight, and smoked like a chimney. His pains led us to do a chest x-ray, which showed unmistakable signs of lung cancer. He needed treatment urgently. We referred him to a Long Island facility that specialized in cases like his, but they didn't have an opening for an uninsured, possibly terminal patient for another eleven months. That's when they scheduled his appointment. Long before the appointment date he died. Could he have lived longer? Most likely.

A Honduran immigrant came to my wife (who is also an ER doctor) with pains in his leg. He was a gardener, and while he was working he'd tripped and fell, but he didn't really know why he'd tripped, or how he had fallen. Tests revealed that he had minimal blood flow to the leg from a leaking abdominal aortic aneurysm. That's when the aorta tears. The man needed surgery immediately. Without it he would die.

The gardener had no insurance, so when a surgeon was asked to look at the case, he refused. I can guess what was going through the surgeon's mind. Working on this patient would be a high-risk, no-pay proposition. We began calling other facilities in a desperate attempt to find a surgeon who would see him. Ten hours later we finally found one, but it was too late. He died in transit to the other facility.

In theory there's a federal law to protect the uninsured in cases like these. The Emergency Medical Treatment and Active Labor Act, or EMTALA, dates from 1973. Congress passed it in reaction to private facilities that made a practice of dumping uninsured patients onto public hospitals. EMTALA guarantees that *anyone* who shows up at any hospital must be given a Medical Screening Exam (MSE) before they are asked about their ability to pay. But what is a Medical Screening Exam? It's an elastic term for diagnosis. A doctor might look at a patient's general appearance, ask a few questions, and take notes on what he sees. Within a few minutes those notes are refined into the patient's MSE. There's no requirement for x-rays, scans, or even a stethoscope. It simply requires that a medical professional take a look, and put a name to what he or she sees.

When you arrive at the ER the first thing you do is sign in. At this point you're usually asked a few questions. This might be considered the MSE, but it's not. Though we're required to do this before asking about payment, these initial questions might also include something about insurance. Once we've established a patient's insurance status, then we have a better idea of the options. Do we have to fight to get the patient to the right doctor, or can that be done with a quick call? Insurance helps determine that.

We've all heard stories about the ER replacing the family doctor for the uninsured. This happens, but it can also become a tool for any doctor who wants tests for a patient. I once worked in the ER of a facility specializing in cardiac cases. Each morning I saw patients who'd been referred to us because they were complaining of chest pains. By the time I saw the patient these chest pains would somehow be gone, but there would always be another problem that appeared to need testing. When I would ask questions it would turn out that their private doctor had instructed the patient to come into the ER complaining of chest pains, but then once the examination began, the patient should say the pains had disappeared. For cardiologists this was a way to jump their patients through all the hoops that stood between them and the always-busy angiogram tables.

All of these practices have a cost and a price. The cost is that of the man-hours, facilities, equipment, and drugs. The more people who work on a patient, the higher the costs. The more tests and treatments, the higher the cost. The longer the patient stays in the hospital, the higher the cost. The more outpatient visits, the higher the cost. As the services mount up, people and institutions need to be paid. The problem is in how they get paid, and that's where price enters the picture.

Every treatment has a price, as does every drug. Many prices are set according to regulations and policies devised by the government, insurers, and the hospitals. Most insurance plans set standard prices they're willing to pay for specific treatments procedure-by-procedure. When insurance plans include prescription drugs, they sometimes cover a percentage, and other times they a set dollar amount. Many plans require druggists to use the least expensive versions (usually generics) of each drug. Some plans do not.

The better insured the patient, the less obstacles to doing whatever might be necessary... or unnecessary. If a fully-insured patient comes in, doctors know they can cover everything. Even if some tests involve copayments, people with comprehensive health plans can almost always afford to pay their share. Doctors also realize that if they don't cover everything with an insured patient they stand a better chance of getting in trouble. Insurers are likely to examine any problem or fault. If a test might conceivably show something that would affect an outcome, the insured patient gets it. If a patient has a hacking cough we might test the heart, lungs, and all other parts of the respiratory system. A well-insured patient with an everyday infection might be tested for everything from cancer to gout, then, when it proves to be nothing but a minor infection, the patient might receive a new and exotic antibiotic at a premium cost.

The more tests we order, the better the chance of false positives. False positives can lead to more tests and/or unnecessary treatments. These tests often lead us into searching for diseases that have no likelihood of being present. We do CAT scans on young people and children who show none of the symptoms that would warrant such a measure, but a false positive result from some other test automatically triggered more testing. I've seen repeated CAT scans done on a patient with a kidney stone, but in the end it was still just a kidney stone. This added to the cost, and to the risk of excess radiation. It added pages to a growing chart. What the extra CAT scans didn't do was add to the patient's wellbeing.

But what if the patient with the minor infection doesn't have insurance? Then if he visits his doctor, the doctor examines him, sees the infection, asks pertinent questions, and prescribes inexpensive penicillin, and the patient pays there and then. What's the difference? The doctor is dealing with an individual rather than an insurance company. There's only so much the patient can pay, so the doctor isn't compelled to do all the extras. Still there are times when more should be done, but the patient can't afford it. If I see something on the x-ray, I have to convince the patient to do it. But if an insurance company, or a government program pays, then further tests are often palatable. If a government program is footing the bill, a doctor wants to check everything. The greater the oversight, the greater the fear that something might be missed. That's why tests can almost always become the justification for more tests.

Insurance plans often cover expensive versions of common drugs. Prices on most of these products and services are usually fixed by insurers, but costs vary widely. When a new miracle drug first hits the market its maker can claim the high cost of development when setting the initial price, but when the drug's been out for several years, does the price go down? Often it doesn't. With many drugs the price remains high until the patent runs out. Then, when facing competition from generic versions, the drug maker might finally cut the price, or might reformulate dosages and schedules to disguise the fact that the price is still the same. Though the drug's actual cost (that of producing and marketing it) doesn't change, the price can change radically from one supplier to another.

The chaotic nature of cost and price in prescription drugs can be seen in this true story of a man and his dog. The dog, a Lab-Shepherd mix, was a victim of Lyme disease. Whenever the pet's owner saw evidence that an attack was in progress, he took the dog to the vet, and she prescribed a two-week course of the antibiotic, doxycycline. Over time the owner got to know these capsules well.

One morning the dog showed the classic symptoms: lethargy, loss of appetite, and stiffness. The owner's wife had taken their car out-of-town that day, making the trip to the vet more difficult. The owner called the vet and asked if doxycycline was ever used for humans, and, if so, could she phone in a prescription to a nearby drugstore. The vet agreed, but said: "I'll have them give you a two-day supply, but bring your dog in tomorrow. I can give you the rest of the prescription here, after I've checked him."

Normally the owner paid the vet just $7 for the course of twenty-eight capsules. There was no insurance involved. That was what the vet charged after putting her standard mark-up on them. At the drugstore they charged him $12 for just four of the caps, twelve times the per-pill rate that the vet charged. When the man asked about it, the druggist simply said: "Sorry. I don't set the prices."

When the dog owner quizzed his vet the next day, she said: "That's why I didn't prescribe the whole course of pills when I called there. I think there are differences in the testing, with tests for humans being a lot more stringent, and that might make the difference, though I'm not really sure."

Hers was the first of numerous vague explanations the owner heard in the coming days, but none of the excuses made much sense. He'd saved one capsule from the drugstore, and it bore the exact same markings as the ones from his vet. How could they tell the tested ones from the untested ones? They couldn't.

This was a case of the simplest explanation being the truth. Testing had nothing to do with it. There was no difference except price. This is confirmed by a study prepared for Congressman Elijah Cummings (D, MD), which reports "that drug manufacturers are engaging in substantial price discrimination, charging low prices for drugs when they are used by animals and high prices for the same drugs when they are used by seniors and other consumers." The study also notes that: "Under the applicable FDA regulations, both human and animal versions of the drugs must meet the same standards for quality and purity." The report blames a pricing structure that eliminates wholesalers from the veterinary sales chain. Manufacturers sell directly to vets, who then sell the drugs to us. [*]

In a few states doctors can sell drugs directly to patients, and some physicians even have vending machines dispensing antibiotics in their waiting rooms. In some of the states that don't allow this, certain specialists are exempted. In my home state of New York doctors can only give out samples of certain drugs—except oncologists. These cancer specialists may sell, dispense and administer in the office. Talk about monopoly!

Wholesaler or no wholesaler, with most products one extra link in the sales chain couldn't explain a twelve-fold discrepancy. Consumer expectations and insurance coverage may also play a role. In the pharmacy we assume we'll pay a lot, so many of us buy insurance with partial or full drug coverage. Drug companies know that most of us will never notice. Few of us get the chance to compare prices the way

---

[*] *Prescription Drug Price Discrimination in the 7th Congressional District of Maryland: Drug Manufacturer Prices Are Higher for Humans than for Animals*, Minority Staff, Special Investigations Division, Committee on Government Reform, U.S. House of Representatives, February 16, 2000, http://www.google.com/url?sa=t&rct=j&q=&esrc=s&source=web &cd=1&ved=0CKoBEBYwAA&url=http%3A%2F%2Fwww.house.g ov%2Fcummings%2Fpdf%2Fanimals.pdf&ei=HiCpT-anEKGf6AGg8Mi9BA&usg=AFQjCNEV25gwfEoiHR2_y0ReJxFuI3r9 2g&sig2=oPYA8Sc4Gc5iscrMgvCpew, accessed 12/15/2011

this man did. It's just one flaw in an incredibly complex system.

Fixing a system like this one isn't easy, but a few principles would provide a good start. Basic healthcare for a healthy person of working age, or for a normal family, should be affordable for any working person. We should pay for checkups and treatments for minor ailments ourselves. Insurance should only cover catastrophic events—heart attacks, cancer, injuries, and other imminent threats to life and limb. Rather than doing every test, no matter how far-fetched the reason, in most situations doctors should be able to describe options, make recommendations, then allow the patient to decide what he or she wants.

For the poor there would still be Medicaid, or something like it, but any government-subsidized health system would be modified. A Medicaid system that requires testing for every contingency, and micromanages every procedure by use of regulations and guidelines, would no longer exist. Instead, Medicaid patients' experiences should be similar to those with private catastrophic insurance who pay for minor ailments. Regulations should be pared down, allowing doctors to describe sensible options. Only then will patients be able to make sensible choices.

Chapter Four: Checks and Balances

Defenders of our health system cite safety as one of the main drivers of higher costs. Other countries don't have the effective regulations we have. We demand that all new drugs be tested, retested, and tested again. We require inspections, safeguards, and security protocols. We build these into every step of research, development, manufacture, and distribution. Whenever questions arise about any drug or treatment, our gut reflex is to take it off the market. This is our system of checks.

If there's one thing modern technology has given us, it's an infinite system of checks. We program these safeguards into every service and transaction. If we exceed our credit limit, we learn it instantly, before the transaction goes through. When we access our private information, programs ask us for our credentials before allowing us in. We design our car dashboards to remind us when our oil is low, or when the radiator needs more water. Software designers put in checks to prevent overloading, and to manage everything from English grammar to nuclear reactions.

We rely on systems to keep us efficient. We count on them to turn the lights on and off, and to funnel rush hour traffic into the correct lanes. We create systems to monitor our honesty, and even our identities. From signatures to fingerprints to iris scans, technology constantly matches who we say we are with its records of who we really are.

Most of us would agree that our most important checks are on safety. We don't trust our systems any more than we trust ourselves. Whenever we set up a new set of security features, we create a second set to check on the first. When both systems break down, we create a third, and so on.

Our first response to most problems is to set up systems to check them, and even repair them before we know anything is wrong. Our first goal in problem-solving always seems to be a solution that covers *all* possible recurrences. We want smooth-running perfection. This isn't just a goal; it's an expectation.

We're great on checks, but checks aren't the same as balances. We forget that modern technology is a fulcrum. On one side we have human needs, on the other, human desires. We all need good health, but we desire complete freedom. We want to feel perfectly fine right now, yet we also want to do fun things that will hurt us later. And we always want someone else to be responsible for any bad outcomes.

Modern medicine can't be perfect. A primary healthcare goal is to preserve life. Lives always end, so our success rate is zero. Another goal is to preserve good health. Good health always either deteriorates, or ends suddenly, so our success rate is zero there too. We do better with short-term goals such as healing fractures and wounds, and curing specific illnesses, but we sometimes miss on these too. Even the world's best doctor has some bad outcomes.

Health is the most obvious and essential quality in any life. When our health is damaged or threatened we go to healthcare professionals. We believe they can cure us, so we demand it. We pay our money, and expect good results. Anything less is their fault, not ours.

Whenever there's a bad outcome doctors, or our surrogates, go back over the treatment. What caused the failure? What could have been done differently? If we spot a flaw, we create a way to check it. If the problem is a sudden change in blood sugar, then we find a way to monitor the change, then a method to double-check the monitor. When an infection sets in, we examine and re-examine our antibiotics regimen, adjusting times and dosages. We then set up new systems to oversee the changes, making sure they are followed every time.

We've all heard of cases where surgeons did the wrong operation on the wrong patient. This seldom happens, but when it does it always makes headlines. The response has been to set up procedures that guarantee five layers of safety in the correct identification of surgical patients. The system works well enough, but is that any better than the old one? The answer is yes, until somehow the system fails again. Then we add even more layers. We believe that every new layer of security is a step toward perfect safety. We believe the impossible.

Those of us who practice modern American medicine are expected to achieve a zero error rate—no mistakes of any kind at any time. Such perfection is a laudable goal, but, like all perfection, it's also impossible. We should always strive to correct mistakes; we should also always remember that, just as dark clouds sometimes have silver linings, medicine occasionally produces happy accidents.

On one crazy night shift Luz Fernandez was admitted to the ER. She was a frail old lady who'd suffered a fall in her home. Ms. Fernandez spoke no English, but my Spanish was good enough to get some of her story. As we talked I began to recognize that this pleasant lady was demented. She explained that she'd fallen out of bed when making her midnight run to the bathroom. She reported that she was suffering back and hip pain after her accident.

I performed a physical and jotted a few notes on her chart, then moved on to my next patients. We had a crowd. A couple of patients later I saw another elderly Hispanic woman who'd arrived, accompanied by her daughter. This one's name was Luz *H*ernandez. Ms. Hernandez's mental capacities were also questionable, and she had a long list of medical concerns. She would need a full evaluation, including blood tests, x-rays and a CAT scan.

As I've said, it was a crazy night even by ER standards. At that frantic pace no one can keep complete control of everything. You simply do your level best, and hope that's enough. Hours rushed by in a blur of patients and problems. Finally, at about three in the morning I was summoned to the phone to speak with our on-duty radiologist.

"What in hell is going on down there?" he asked.

"Bedlam," I said. "What do you have for me?"

"You've got a large sub-dural hematoma* on that elderly woman who fell."

"You mean the lady with the mental status changes? Hernandez?"

"Not her," he said, "*Fernandez*, not *Hernandez*."

I squeezed my eyes shut, trying to remember which letter went with which woman's name. "But I didn't order a CT on *Fernandez*," I said, "or maybe... "

As we tried to sort it out, it began to look as if I'd ordered the CT on the wrong patient. At least, at that moment I thought she was the wrong patient. But as the radiologist went into more detail, and I shook off the confusion of the night's pandemonium, I realized I'd somehow done right, even though I'd meant to do something else that might've had more negative consequences. They'd

---

* Blood on the brain.

done the CT on Ms. *F*ernandez, which wasn't what I'd intended, and they'd discovered a huge issue no one had even suspected was there: the hematoma. She went straight to the neurosurgeons, who successfully operated on her.

Meanwhile I put in a new order for the CT on Ms. *H*ernandez. The results came back negative. Ms. *F*ernandez's family was grateful, and they believed I must be a magician. I'd found the problem no one else had detected. I smiled and went about my night believing in medicine, luck and fortune. I probably should've picked up a few lottery tickets on my way home.

If our attitude toward mistakes is unrealistic, and often counterproductive, our notion of checks and balances is even more skewed. As we devise ever more checks we tend to completely ignore balances. When we invent a machine that can test for a disease, we first test it on an incredibly narrow set of patients with obscenely rigid criteria. Only those who have the best chance of benefit get this. Only when we get an outcome with potential for both benefit and profitability, do we expand it, and then we tend to expand it to everyone. We set some obvious limits, usually for age, sex, or pre-existing conditions, but, staying true to our first instinct, we test as broad a range of patients as possible, even those whose chances of getting the disease are almost nil. This is where balances should return us to sanity. A sensible approach would balance the test's potential to detect threats, along with the patient's symptoms and history, against the real costs in money and time.

Checks cost money. In any normal system, that alone would bring balance into the process. If someone has to monitor a surgeon to insure that he uses the right equipment, that person has to be paid. If the check is mechanical, money pays for the machine, its development, and its operation. In either case the check takes time. These safeguards are easy to begin but hard to stop.

Hospitals have a process called CQI—Continuous Quality Improvement. CQI is an examination of the processes to insure that standards for quality care are met. Are the hospital's standard procedures leading to the desired outcomes? If not, should the procedures be altered? If so, how? Most hospitals have groups or committees who meet once a month to measure these. These groups review cases and analyze errors. When there's been a bad outcome, the hospital does a Root Cause Analysis, or RCA. The RCA analyzes the process, examines the procedure, and then the thinking behind the procedure, until it gets to the root cause. Once that's identified, the hospital modifies the process to change the end. The solution is seldom proactive. Instead of changing what's already there, the hospital officials usually add another check to the system—another safety measure.

This is how doctors protect themselves. As long as someone or some system is checking them, they can fall back on that. If an error happens the fault is in the checks. The way to stop it is to add more checks. These checks do more to protect doctors than patients.

In most cases doctors control costs. We are the ones who pay the premiums for malpractice insurance. We are the ones who administer the tests, then call for more tests. Our demands drive a medical industry that is always devising more testing instruments to meet our demands. We take the instruments and devise new testing protocols. We advertise safety and testing on TV and in other media. Along with this comes a drug industry that advertises new prescription antidotes for every ailment. Viewers see these new drugs and procedures through the smiling faces of attractive patients, and they want the same for themselves—but they want complete safety too. We pretend this is possible. We encourage the irrational.

Until doctors adopt a rational approach to this unchecked system of checks medical prices will go up, but that won't happen until our fear of litigation goes down. Until patients adopt rational expectations, prices will go up. But how can we change patient expectations when doctors and drug companies make their products look like panaceas? The system is based on false premises: infinite care, infinite drugs, and infinite positive outcomes. As long as the foundation is false, anything built on it is likely to be just as false. If doctors controlled their costs, and patients paid fair prices for rational treatments and procedures, American medicine would look very different—and better. But we would have to give up our idea that every process must be completely safe, and that our ability to cure is infinite.

We always have good reasons to introduce safety measures. Usually the main drivers are cases that end in bad outcomes. We react to the unexpected death, the operation on the wrong patient, or the procedure that went tragically haywire. The case is analyzed, the problem identified, and a safety measure is introduced to solve it. When the safeguard is new everyone repeats the story of its cause. Soon this story becomes an instructional tool. Whenever the new measure is used, we note the juncture where things went wrong, and watch the process go right. The safeguard works every time, leaving us with the impression that every time a check occurs, a serious error has been averted. Though it looks that way, it's almost never true. If the error occurred 1% of the time, then that's probably how often the safeguard prevents it. 99% of the time the error would never come up.

We tend to be all-or-nothing in our thinking. If something bad happens some of the time, we want a total solution—one that keeps the bad thing from ever happening again. We want to identify and solve all problems before they have any consequences. We regard every bad outcome as a complete failure to be avoided at all costs—no matter who pays. In American medicine our goal has become a zero error rate. When we diagnose an illness we should be right every time. The most complex operations should always work flawlessly. Therapies should always lead to good results. A drug, when properly prescribed and taken, should always do as advertised.

If we can't afford the infinite, we assume our insurance company can. And therein lies another root of fallacy.

Chapter Five: Rationality and Rationing

Healthcare is rationed. It is now, it always has been, and it always will be. The village healer tends to the chief before treating the village bum. In the old South the plantation owner received a doctor's best efforts, while the slave made do with primitive home remedies. The same is true today. The criterion isn't always money. Sometimes it's simply proximity to research facilities where the newest treatments are being tested. Other times it's the quality of one's coverage.

The makers of the film, *John Q*, explored the question of limitations on healthcare in a life-and-death situation. The movie tells the story of a little boy needing a heart transplant. When he's denied the operation due to financial constraints, his father takes the occupants of an operating room hostage, threatening to harm them if his son is left to die. This is the ultimate nightmare stemming from rationed care. It is dramatic, horrific and intolerable. It is also inevitable.

When a life hangs in the balance rationing can push anyone to the breaking point, but what happens when the rationing is applied to large populations? What might be the best-known case of healthcare rationing in history is that of penicillin. The antibiotic was first discovered in 1928, yet throughout the 1930s it remained unavailable to the general public. Funding for experiments testing treatments and production methods was almost nonexistent in the midst of the Great Depression. World War II changed that. Allied governments got serious about research in 1940. By 1942 with wars raging on two fronts, the U.S. produced small test batches. Finally, in 1943 we began producing the drug on a large scale. Still, in the war years there was never enough. The first doses went to the military, with any excess going to civilians. In the last two years of the war penicillin saved thousands of servicemen's lives and limbs, but in some field hospitals, and back here in the States, patients who might've lived were still dying. The government called it "allocation of resources," but its real name was: rationing.

In the postwar years production in the U.S. increased to the point where most Americans could get it with reasonable ease. Our doctors began prescribing it freely. But an impoverished, war-ravaged Europe received little. That's the key to the plot of another famous movie, *The Third Man.* The classic film is set in post-World War II Vienna. A crime lord schemes to control the city's tiny ration of penicillin. The moviegoers of 1949 understood the problem. Stories like that in the film were making the headlines every day.

Penicillin was the ultimate wonder drug. It was the first, and most visible, of the long line of antibiotics that changed medicine in the postwar years. In most patients it could kill an infection, or prevent one from starting. It made surgery far less dangerous, and successfully treated millions for conditions that had once spelled almost certain death. It and its sister drugs became the most essential factor in longevity increases in the last half of the 20th century. With most users, it wasn't just a pill that kept them barely alive. Most of those who lived longer due to antibiotics also lived well.

Yet in those first years after the War penicillin went only to the lucky and/or the rich. If you needed it, money and proximity ruled your fate. It happened in Europe, Japan, China, and right here in the USA. As they allocated limited supplies governments, institutions and individual doctors had to decide who got it and who didn't. This triage was life-and-death rationing on a massive scale. People didn't like it, but they resigned themselves to reality until supplies increased.

Rationing is still with us, and will continue to be as long as we keep making advances in medicine. Whenever a new, life-saving drug or procedure becomes available, it's limited. If a doctor devises a new surgical method, it's rationed to his patients, with all others excluded. As he trains more doctors, and they train others, more patients get it. But as long as some patients can get it, while others can't, the method is rationed. The same is true for new drugs and new therapies. Government and institutional regulations limit the use of new medicines and treatments until they've been proven effective. Safety is also an issue. Materials, methods, and skills are rationed by time, training, and production capacity. All of these things require money, so finance always plays a part.

Insurers and healthcare providers never say this. In the public mind rationing is a dirty word when applied to medicine. In the first debates about Medicare in the 1940s "rationing" was mentioned only in the context of withholding care in medical emergencies. The term gained an immoral odor, as if any limitation on a doctor's time or resources was a crime. Ever since then, that's how we've seen the whole issue of allocated care. When today's policymakers address healthcare, rationing remains the ultimate taboo. Public plans are always scrutinized for instances of rationing. Private insurers avoid the word entirely, hiding the necessary practice in any way they can. But if we want to allow medicine to advance, we must tolerate the inevitable rationing. Otherwise none of us will receive any new drug or treatment—ever.

A recent example of widespread rationing on a nationwide scale was the flu vaccine shortage of 2009. That fall the United States found itself with a higher demand for flu vaccine, but less doses to give out. This situation grew from public policy and individual expectations. Throughout the last couple of decades more and more of us have been getting flu shots. Many of us consider the vaccine to be a basic part of our health regimen, but American drug companies have been increasingly reluctant to manufacture it. Government policies limit what manufacturers can charge, while failing to adequately protect them from patients' lawsuits. This situation sent most vaccine production overseas. In 2009 some foreign producers allocated more for other buyers, including their own governments and citizens. This left us with far fewer doses just as demand was peaking. Providers and regulators had to decide who got it and who didn't.

In a less constrained environment, where reasonable profits were allowed, and where manufacturers felt safe from the threat of bankrupting legal actions, there would have been enough. In that kind of atmosphere American companies would be free to make and market the vaccine properly. Instead we accept shortages, forcing real rationing of effective vaccines that should be readily available. But we never use the word.

In the case of a vaccine we can avoid facing the fact of rationing by emphasizing the shortage that caused it. It shouldn't have happened. This wasn't experimentation or research. It was a known quantity that was already being produced at a predictable cost. The shortage was simply a mistake in planning—a scandal of incompetence. When officials proposed ways to avoid the problem in the future, their main concern was creating more backup systems: fail-safe production schedules with the potential to manufacture far more doses than would ever be necessary. Three years later, with the shortage slipping beyond memory, and every

Walmart and Target pharmacy in the nation offering on-the-spot flu shots each fall, few even recall there was ever a problem. If a thousand extra deaths stemmed from flu complications one winter, that's long past. The situation was temporary, the suffering was unfortunate, but now all is well. But there's one area where rationing is a permanent reality: organ transplants, like the one in *John Q*.

Up until the mid-20th century most transplants were the stuff of science fiction. One of the biggest factors in changing that was the production of antibiotics noted above. This made any surgery safer, opening the way for medical researchers to experiment with transplanting human organs. In the postwar era, as scientists devised drugs to control rejection, some transplants passed from experimentation into practice.

Ever since the early successes in the 1950s and 1960s, transplants have been publicized, sensationalized, and scrutinized. In the late-20th century, as medicine solved many of the problems of organ rejection, some types of transplants became commonplace. Thousands of kidneys and livers are transplanted every year, but there are never enough. In the United States in 2010 there were 112,000 patients waiting for transplants, but only 22,104 organs actually went from one body to another.* Four out of five patients either died, or found some other way to survive the year.

If you've ever known anyone awaiting a transplant you've seen life-and-death rationing in action. The patient waits, and if the wait goes on too long, the patient dies. This suspense creates anxiety, depression, and worse. When an organ becomes available, that information goes onto various

---

* Statistics from http://www.donatelifeny.org/about-donation/data/#Data%20US1, accessed 12/23/2011.

lists around the world. The lists include organs from a particular area or population, and patients who are waiting for them. Though there are ethical and legal barriers to using net worth as a criterion for selecting patients, wealth does play a role. Ability to pay is still a qualification, so you must have either access to cash, or the proper insurance coverage. Those with the best coverage usually have more wealth, and the wealthy have the time and resources to get themselves on more lists worldwide. If an organ is suddenly available in India, it takes ready cash to pay for the overnight plane ticket necessary to go claim the prize. As long as many patients are chasing few resources some variation of this process will ration distribution.

So though we may deny the existence of rationing, we accept its practice in everything from a bout with the flu to a brand new heart. Medicine is a product like any other. Though it can twist and disguise its relationship to the laws of supply-and-demand, it can't entirely avoid them. The first ones who line up with the money are usually the first ones to get the product.

This isn't an argument for basing all decisions about drug manufacturing on profit alone. Products essential to life and good health shouldn't be entirely governed by everyday business practices. Still, qualified private sector companies must be allowed to charge a realistic price, with the assurance that they won't face legal actions for competent, good faith efforts. In the case of the flu vaccine such policies could have eliminated the need for rationing in the U.S. With other, less plentiful pharmaceuticals, if we were to make a straightforward admission of the need to ration, we would see the problem more clearly, which would allow us to make more effective policies. Those policies would ration drugs to those with the most need (thus with the highest real demand).

We hate the idea of rationing because we accept the false notions of unlimited insurance benefits and endless healthcare resources. Our individual and national attitudes about healthcare allocation (rationing) are based on three insane premises. The first is that healthcare is infinite. When it comes to health, Americans like to be optimists. "Where there's life there's hope," we tell ourselves, and no matter how bleak the prognosis, we hang onto our hope for miracles, and/or sudden medical advances. This expectation of infinite healthcare options allows no room for death. In the end the only positive outcome is immortality.

The second premise is that all patients are equal, so all treatments should be equal too. If two patients have similar cancers, and one gets the brand new anti-cancer drug, the other should get it too. If there's only enough for one needy cancer victim, something is terribly wrong. After all, if we were to take this equality one small step further, giving the drug to one patient would deny it to the other, so the only possible solutions would be to either increase supply (which we've already assumed to be impossible), or take the drug out of the equation. With it gone at least both patients could die with clear consciences.

The third premise is that every patient should expect to have access to every existing beneficial drug and treatment, no matter how expensive. As long as we pay our insurance premiums, we should get everything—the latest drugs, the most up-to-date therapies, and consultations with the best brains in the business. But what if the cure is only available in some other country? And what if your health policy only covers treatments and drugs here in the U.S.? Then the cure goes to some other patient, and we have rationing once again. We just don't admit it.

The worst way to deal with rationing is to deny it, but denial is our national policy. This leads to ignorance even among policymakers. When faced with the fact of more patients than there are doses, we respond with convenient fictions. Most vaccine manufacturers are overseas, we say, ignoring the fact that this stems from our ruinous legal and regulatory environment. We tell ourselves that these foreign producers violate their contracts, and withhold our vaccine, but we never consider that they may be obligated to sell to their own citizens first, or that their other customers might be willing to pay a price based on the real cost. We view these issues through the lens of our own needs and desires, and the status quo. How can we change something so complex, and so dependent on foreign companies? We should consider ways to solve the problem ourselves.

To do that we would have to admit that the problem is here in our own country. We would need to accept that any solution must happen here, or not happen at all. We would have to look at why we don't make enough vaccine in America. Once we accepted the truth, we would find ourselves facing difficult choices on politically taboo topics. We would be unable to escape the fact that our medical supply system is based on the false notions that we can provide an infinite amount of care and medicine, and that the only issues are the affordability of insurance premiums, and who will actually pay for medical care.

A complete health system would be based on the fact that "complete" is an evolving concept with built-in limitations. There is no infinite supply of drugs, therapies or other treatments. There is only what's available at an affordable price to the patient. The price must be set according to the cost of provision. If prices were set on the basis of real cost, with a standard markup, as they are in other businesses, most medical problems would be affordable even to those on average incomes. In most cases we would pay when we receive the service, or, if the price is truly beyond our means, and the service is necessary, our insurance provider would pay for whatever our policy covers. If the service isn't covered, and we don't have the resources to pay, then we might be in a situation where we simply can't afford it. At that point we must discuss realistic alternatives with our doctor. These might not be exactly what we want or need. That's a reality we hide from, but we must learn to accept it. In any of these scenarios, price should be an accurate reflection of cost, along with a reasonable profit.

We avoid the idea of rationing because we don't want to see medicine as a business. We want medicine and altruism to go hand-in-hand, just as we dream of every doctor being like Marcus Welby: a wise and gallant knight of the profession. Doctors are supposed to be healers, and in our minds healers must adhere to a code that lies outside the crass concerns of money. But in the years since Welby went off the air, our rosy ideas about medicine have been rocked by one headline after another. The malpractice crisis of the late 1970s put chinks in the knightly armor. The cost of insurance, procedures and drugs took medicine down a few more notches in public consciousness. Scandals in hospitals, pharmaceutical companies, and other healthcare institutions tarnished the image further. Reports of everything from misdiagnoses to surgeries done on the wrong patients, have left the public's perception of the medical profession in tatters. We think of medical ethics as something that has to be restored.

Doctors have reacted with understandable fear and caution. If you see a competent colleague fulfilling all of his duties, yet a patient sues him for failing to recommend a certain test, you begin calling for the same test, no matter how improbable the risk might be. Once a test is covered by basic insurance, you do it even if it seems unnecessary.

When CAT scans became available patients wanted them. These scans would catch the tumors doctors had missed. When MRIs were developed, reducing radiation risks, and increasing the accuracy of images, patients wanted those instead. In both cases the technology was expensive at first, then became much more reasonable as the number of machines, and personnel trained to use them, increased. In both cases, once insurance companies covered the procedures, patients demanded them, and many doctors and hospitals promoted them. Did your head ache? Were you getting pains in your chest or your stomach? Was it cancer? Was a heart attack imminent? Was it possible that you'd had a stroke? Even if the chances were one-in-a-million, why ignore the risk? Here was technology that could look inside, and show you every bump and node, and somewhere some faceless entity would pay for it.

This gave the public the impression that we could detect every tumor before it grew, and every microbe before it multiplied. If you had a symptom that might possibly go with some type of cancer, we could look, and find out for sure. (But was it really for sure? None of these tests are fail-safe, so many tests are backed up by other tests. The more testing you do the more false positives you get, and that drives the need for more testing. Though few admit it, miss rates on diagnoses are often just as high for the machines as they are for doctors who simply look, listen and touch.) As the tests grew more common, more doctors called for them. As more patients got them, even more patients wanted them. As the price became affordable, more policies paid for them. Once this was true, the price settled at an amount that covered the actual cost of the imaging, then added ample payments for everyone in the process. Anyone who had a function in the scanning process also had a stake in the payments. Doctors, technicians, administrators, hospitals, sales people, and manufacturers all shared the wealth. We invented, developed, and preserved this system, and it rules American healthcare today.

A CAT scan might be $275, with an MRI going for $800. The doctor might recommend the less expensive test, but the patient with coverage might demand the pricier one. Why not? Insurance will pay for it. With research, development, and marketing costs already paid, the provider can give the test for a cost of just a few dollars. In any other business the price would drop with the cost, but this isn't any business. This is our health we're talking about. That's why we have insurance. We need a source of endless money to pay for endless options. We want to be able to pay whatever amount it takes to stay alive and healthy—or even just alive.

Though the truth can set us free, sometimes it requires payment. If we base our decisions on the truth, we can learn real costs, set sensible prices, and get better healthcare for that payment.

Chapter Six: Insurance

There are many different kinds of insurance. Most insurance isn't required by law, but almost all insurance is legally regulated. We think of insurance as a measure of responsibility, and in many cases it is. One of our yardsticks for evaluating responsibility behind the wheel is the driver's choice of insurance policies. We wouldn't think to criticize a parent of young children who buys life insurance. When we get a mortgage on a house, the mortgage provider requires insurance against fire, and various other physical threats. When we've paid off the mortgage it's wise to keep up that insurance even though no law forces us to. For most of us the house is our biggest investment.

Health insurance is unique. If it's going to work we must create sensible definitions of good health and bad health, then examine treatments, procedures, and materials to find out what costs what. Two consumers might shop for insurance with the same goal: coverage that will pay the bills to keep them healthy. One might find it reasonable to want insurance against every sniffle. The other might feel perfectly fine with a policy that doesn't kick in until the life-threatening heart attack. Insurers have many policies in many price ranges for both.

In America health insurance began in the early 20th century, evolving out of earlier policies aimed at accidents and their resulting disabilities. In the Great Depression of the 1930s, when so many patients couldn't pay for services on the spot, doctors and patients joined in insurance programs that allowed patients to pay regularly scheduled premiums, and receive the care they needed. This simple arrangement was something like insurance, and something like an installment plan. Doctors received limited payments on time, and patients knew what bills would be due when. Many states' Blue Cross and Blue Shield insurance programs grew from these efforts. In those days medicine was simpler, costs were lower, and limitations were clearer. There was only so much a doctor or hospital could do. People accepted that.

After World War II medicine grew. With the advent of the antibiotics, vaccines, and miracle technologies we've talked about, the medical profession could help millions of patients who'd once been condemned to misery or death. As antibiotics dramatically lowered the risk of infection, and miniaturization made the use of tools like lasers and radiation more precise, procedures no one had even thought possible became routine. All of this cost money—more money than most individuals could afford to pay at one time.

In the postwar years health insurance became a basic tenet in our idea of the good life. Americans wanted a nice home, a good car, the best educations possible for their children, and plenty of leisure. If we were going to enjoy this ideal to its fullest we needed one more thing: good health. But some of the greatest advances in medicine cost more than even a well-to-do American could pay. Health insurance seemed like a sensible solution—and it worked.

Prodded by wartime austerity measures, health insurance had already expanded to much of the American work force. During World War II, with 16 million Americans serving in the armed forces, manufacturers faced severe labor shortages, and both employers and unions had to follow wartime regulations capping wages. Companies competing for labor were hamstrung in what they could offer prospective workers in their pay envelopes. Union leaders faced the same limitations. Once they reached the government-mandated wage ceilings, they couldn't ask for more. When they met to sort out new labor contracts what could negotiators do? One solution was fringe benefits—employer-paid services not included in wage rates. These could guarantee workers certain features of the good life without running afoul of Washington.

First they went for pension funds so any union member could retire at 65. The pensions, supplemented by the brand new Social Security system, would guarantee that retired employees could live reasonably well, and avoid becoming drains on their children's resources. Once unions had made progress on workers' old age benefits, health was next. Workers in many industries began to receive health insurance packages for themselves, and often for their families. In the second half of the 20th century this practice spread beyond the unionized workforce, and eventually a majority of working Americans got their health insurance from their jobs.

As soon as people began paying a simple, steady premium (often deducted before they ever saw their paycheck) their expectations began to rise. They wanted that premium to cover everything. Policies began paying for much more than the calamities of illness and accident. Insured patients got lower and lower deductibles. Often even their routine check-ups were covered, sometimes fully, other times with a small copayment from the patient. Doctors and insurance providers encouraged this, promoting the coverage of routine healthcare as "preventative medicine." This was based on the notion that the routine examinations would find warning signs before they became real problems.

Patients with insurance from work usually went only to doctors and hospitals that accepted their policies. Insurance providers negotiated with hospitals and physicians' groups to keep prices low for their policyholders. If these policyholders went to doctors outside the system, they often found higher prices, and these usually weren't covered by their policies. By the late 1960s uninsured patients who fell below the poverty line often qualified for federal and state Medicaid programs. Working poor with no job-based benefits fell through the cracks. The assumption was that, given half a chance, these patients would skip out on their bills. The solution was to charge patients without coverage far more, and collect as many fees as possible at the door. This resulted in the working uninsured paying the highest prices of all. In other words, if you were uninsured and poor, but not poor enough, you paid three, four, or five times the price that an insured patient paid for the same treatment. This was one major step in the separation of price from real cost.

These private and public programs also made for a less personal medical system. Insured patients had to go to doctors who participated in their company or union health plan. If the insurance changed, often your doctor changed too. Many patients had little choice in this, and even those who could choose faced an extra layer of bureaucracy whenever they made a change. Patients and healthcare providers had more forms to fill out, and more regulations to follow. Red tape often seemed to trump real people. By this time, like Elvis, Dr. Welby had left the building.

This gap between doctors and patients was one factor in an overall decline in the public's respect for the medical profession. That decline played a part in the sudden explosion of malpractice suits in the 1970s. The suits led to doctors being compelled to pay huge premiums for malpractice insurance. That forced many physicians in private practice to combine into much larger practices with other doctors. Being in a large group helped defray some of their insurance costs, but it also added to the impersonal factor. If your doctor wasn't available you were often referred to someone else. As long as a patient's insurance still covered just about everything, he or she tended to accept the change.

In the last few decades this system has grown exponentially, with little or no control. The system itself is a slave to our expectations. When we ask for the infinite, the system tries to give it to us. When the infinite is unaffordable the system juggles the cost-price equation, automatically searching for ways to give us all we want, with no thought to financial consequences. But money is always finite, as are its sources.

Insurance is always a bet between you and your insurer. Each billing period you gamble a few hundred dollars that your house will burn, collapse or be burgled. Your insurance company bets that it won't. Because the house and possessions will cost many thousands to repair or replace, your insurer needs to win that bet far more often than not, or go out of business. After all, if the people with intact homes and possessions drop their policies, who's going to pay? For decades this has been a primary problem in health insurance: many healthy people, particularly among the young, don't want to bet that they'll get sick. In the short run most of them are right. In the long run almost all are wrong. So how do we get the uninsured to buy health policies?

In the mid-20th century another type of insurance emerged that dealt with the problem of the willfully uninsured. It's the coverage we have on our cars. In the same years when medicine was transforming itself into one of our major industries, the automobile came to dominate America's landscape. Americans' desire to drive was every bit as strong as our desire for good health, but when we got out on the highway we tended to crash at alarming rates. We wrecked our cars, and mangled our bodies, running up incredible bills. Mechanics and doctors had their work cut out for them, and someone had to pay.

The solution most states adopted was legislation requiring drivers to have minimum liability insurance (MLI). You could buy a car without it, but if you drove that car on your state's public roads you had to buy an inexpensive minimal insurance package. These minimum packages didn't do much for you or your car. If you got hurt, or your car was totaled, the responsibility was yours. You paid your mechanic and your doctor—or your estate did. But the MLI did cover the valid claims of anyone you ran into. The idea was that you could do whatever damage you wanted to yourself and your car, and you would have to deal with the consequences, but if you crashed into someone else, they wouldn't have to pay for your irresponsibility.

Massachusetts passed the first of these laws in 1925. For over thirty years they were the only state to make this insurance compulsory. Finally in 1956 New York followed suit. In the '60s and '70s almost all the other states did the same. Today New Hampshire is the only place in the U.S. without such a law. The "Live Free or Die" state relies on a statute requiring drivers to prove they can pay minimal damages before registering their car. Most of the other forty-nine states adopted the minimum liability solution because it had proved itself in Massachusetts and New York. It doesn't solve every problem, but it's been a workable policy.

Healthcare policymakers would do well to adapt this model to medical insurance. It solves the problem of a vast pool of uninsured healthy people without forcing these reluctant consumers to buy today's expensive full-coverage policies. The Patient Protection and Affordable Care Act (PPACA) of 2010 (often called Obamacare) contained a requirement for all citizens to have full health coverage, but that has become the most controversial aspect of a controversial law. It's been declared constitutional, but many would like to see its repeal. Even if it survives, its functionality remains open to question.

The writers of PPACA knew that healthy, uninsured people won't be healthy forever. At some point we all get sick or injured. As a society we aren't comfortable with turning away the needy at the ER door, so these uninsured will be treated somewhere somehow. That means someone has to pay. If we can't force these future patients to buy health insurance, what can we do?

The solution is health insurance stripped down to its most essential elements: a minimum liability policy. Every citizen who could pay would be required to buy a policy that covered catastrophic accidents and illnesses. These policies would not cover checkups, or even most tests, but if you were ill or injured to the point where you needed more expensive medical care than you could reasonably afford, your MLI policy would cover you.

Health insurance isn't auto insurance, so the process wouldn't be exactly the same. For drivers MLI is always for the other guy. When legislators passed bills establishing MLI for drivers they weren't worried about what you do to your own body or car. They were worried about everyone around you. The insurance is for your victims, not for you. The health equation is different. If you're injured or ill, you are the primary victim. You are the one who needs coverage. You are the one whose financial health is in jeopardy. But is it just you?

Here it gets more complex. Other victims aren't immediately obvious, but they are there. The other victims are all of us: insured patients, taxpayers, charitable funds, and so on. If you don't buy insurance, but then you fall ill with a million-dollar disease, we don't slam the ER door on you. We admit you, and treat you as well as we can with whatever modern medicine has to offer. You might not have a private room with five-star hotel-style service, but we'll deal with your immediate problems, and set out a course of treatment aimed at curing you, or at least keeping you alive, no matter what the cost.

But if the cost is of no concern, who pays? Everyone. The hospital pays for staff, supplies, equipment, maintenance, and other items. This becomes a factor in prodding hospital administrators to set higher prices, often across the board. Some of the price rise is paid by insurance companies, who pass the cost on to their policyholders. That means you, me, and millions of others, many of whom get their policies through their jobs. The same applies to any wealthy patient paying cash for services. That patient's bill rises along with all the others. As prices for private insurance go up, so do prices for public coverage. Unpaid bills subtract from hospital revenues. When this shows up in a shrinking bottom line, all those who pay will pay more, including Medicare, Medicaid, and all other public sources.

If you wreck someone's car, and you can't pay for the repairs, the other guy has to. Maybe he has insurance for this, or maybe he doesn't, but you've passed the buck to him. If you get cancer, but you can't pay for treatment, no other individual is likely to pay for you. The government might. A nonprofit might. Or maybe the hospital will absorb some of the cost. Whoever pays, the bill ultimately comes back to the rest of us. We pay it in higher taxes, higher premiums, or we might even give it voluntarily through a charitable organization. In many cases a non-paying patient benefits from all these resources. Each case is different. One patient might get Medicaid, while another patient can't qualify. The uninsured patient might attend a church, or be a member of an organization, with programs that benefit needy members. Some patients qualify for local government programs, while others might receive help from charitable sources. The vagueness and variability of these sources plays into the hands of a system that's out of control. The one constant is that someone or some entity always pays.

That means we pay. It'll be there in the checks we write for taxes and insurance. It's there in the dollars we put in the collection basket at church. It could be a part of our dues to a union or organization, or, more directly, in a healthcare bill not covered by our insurance. But, whatever route the money might take, we can't escape paying it. We foot the bill for the uninsured.

If we hold to the parallel with car insurance, we're the victims in this accident. When the employed, but uninsured, patient who doesn't qualify for Medicaid, has a health smash-up, we're all like the insured driver on the other end of the crash. The uninsured guy ran a red light, plowed right into us, and when they test his blood it'll show up as 90 proof. Yet there he goes in the ambulance, and we're left holding the bag. In healthcare we seldom even know we're crashing, because this smashup leaves thousands of victims. Each pays just a few cents toward the bills of the injured party, but those cents add up. After all, tens of millions of healthy folks are uninsured.

Every comprehensive healthcare proposal has had to deal with healthy people who don't want insurance. But how is this different from the driver that doesn't want insurance? Until he or she has an accident the issue is dormant. And maybe—just maybe—that driver will go a lifetime accident-free. It's theoretically possible. But how many people never have a health problem? For all intents and purposes, not one.

Even the healthy guy who proudly professes that he's never been to a doctor is almost certainly forgetting a few things. Was he born at home, with no healthcare professional present? Did he receive any vaccinations as a child? And as for his future needs: when he breaks a leg, or collapses with a heart attack, will he still refuse treatment? Is he willing to die rather than allow the healthcare system to heal him?

We're all in this together. Even if your only healthcare transactions are for band-aids or aspirin, you're participating in the system. If you're willing to accept treatment for a wound, break, or illness you're dependent on the system. And if you're willing to accept treatment, then you should also be willing to pay. No individual can know what his or her future healthcare will cost, but when the time comes, that cost must be covered. This isn't just an individual issue because we're all affected. It's like our roads: we will all use this system sometime, so we must all share the cost. The alternative would be a system that demands cash at the door. If you came in on a gurney, but didn't have proven means to pay, the hospital would turn you away. It would be similar to the uninsured driver who abandons his smashed up car, but in this case the abandoned item is a human being.

In the world of cars they've stripped down insurance to its barest minimums: you have to pay for the damage you cause to other people and things. In healthcare we should each have to pay for the illnesses and injuries that happen to our bodies. If our maladies are caused by others, we might be able to get them to pay, but either way, the initial responsibility for dealing with the bills should be the individual's. We can achieve this by designing minimum liability policies. The deductible should be quite high—in the thousands at least, and possibly the low five figures. Coverage should only be for expensive procedures and treatments that are not elective. If you need emergency bypass surgery or chemotherapy, you pay your deductible, then your MLI policy kicks in. If you want a nose job, you pay the whole bill.

As in auto insurance, each state could devise its own methods. Just as many states copied the Massachusetts model for MLI, successful state minimum health insurance programs would draw imitators. If the present administration had used an MLI model for Obamacare, the PPACA might not face attempts at repeal—and it wouldn't cost anywhere near as much.

The operative principle would be about the same: If you're an able-bodied American with a job or assets, and you're going to use the roads, breathe the air and drink the water, then you must take responsibility for the cost of keeping your body healthy.

Chapter Seven: Health and Taxes

Who are the uninsured? Most aren't the poorest. Less than a quarter of the uninsured are below the poverty level. These are people who qualify for Medicaid and other public programs, but haven't signed up for them.

While they aren't in dire poverty, most of the uninsured aren't wealthy either. The vast majority are working poor. They get regular paychecks, lifting their incomes above the poverty line, but they are still well below average by any measure. About 30 million of them, or roughly two-thirds, have incomes equivalent to under $44,000 for a family of four.

If there were a typical uninsured family of four, ineligible for Medicaid, it might look like this: two wage earners, each working an average of 30 hours a week (many are sporadically unemployed, or work jobs with limited and/or irregular hours), for an average of $12 per hour. This couple has two dependent children and a total pre-tax income of just over $37,000 per year. For this family the $3,000-to-$4,000 per year for just one minimum coverage policy covering one family member is unaffordable. If we extend this minimal coverage to a spouse and children, the price goes from unaffordable to literally impossible.

Many of the uninsured are children, who have no choice in the matter, but 43% (nearly 20 million) are working-age adults who lack coverage, and make more than 2.5 times poverty-level income.[*] Some of those lacking coverage are single or childless, and should be able to afford

---

[*] From The New York Times editorial, "The Uninsured," August 22, 2009.

high-deductible catastrophic policies. So why don't they buy them?

We usually think of those who won't pay for health insurance as deadbeats, and certainly some of them are. Someone who has a reasonably good job should take the responsibility to get insurance against medical catastrophe. If the job comes with the offer of voluntary health benefits, and the person doesn't take advantage of them, that's even more irresponsible. But most of the uninsured aren't in this kind of situation. Many work in jobs that don't offer health insurance of any kind. 54.2% of them have a high school education or less. Only 16.8% have graduated from college.[**] Obviously the less educated will have less income, so more of them will lack healthcare coverage, but income isn't the only factor. Often someone who's deciding whether or not to enter the system is more afraid of complexity than of price. No one wants to pay for more red tape, but consumers shopping for health coverage usually know: that's exactly what they are doing.

Almost all of us who have insurance have dealt with the healthcare bureaucracies. Some are public, others are private, but all have forms, questionnaires, regulations, and other mountains of paperwork. Government, hospitals, and insurance companies are all in the business of collecting data. Much of it is personal information of a kind we seldom share with anyone but close friends and family. Though we're usually assured that our privacy isn't being violated, giving up any privacy protections is never comfortable, and often feels downright threatening. This is especially true for those at the low end of the financial ladder. Perhaps the most obvious parallel is one that applies to many of the same,

---

[**] http://www.rwjf-eriu.org/fastfacts/cps2005_7.html, accessed 2/14/12.

uninsured citizens: the tax code. A high proportion of the uninsured get paid under-the-table. They avoid 1040s the same way they sidestep insurance forms—they stay away from the entire system. When they do go on the tax rolls they accept withholding, file EZ forms for their refunds, but otherwise remain below the government's radar. To them bureaucracy is always threatening.

America's health and taxation systems grew up in tandem. Both really got going in the early 1900s, giving them a full century to grow into the monsters they are today. Both involve huge amounts of money, a ton of regulations, incalculable waste and countless special interests. Both have been subject to constant tinkering, but attempts at total overhaul have been rare and unsuccessful. They are huge, incredibly complex labyrinths that defy rational explanation. In both systems, complexity combines with necessity, making them almost impervious to change. When small change— or even big change—does occur, it usually increases the complications, wrapping the whole system in one more spool of thick red tape. Witness the overhaul of income taxes in 1985, or the new maze created by the healthcare legislation of 2010. One hugely popular original aim of both proposals was to simplify the bureaucratic process for the average citizen. In both cases this goal was the first to be jettisoned.

As long as someone is healthy, he or she can avoid doctors and hospitals, and most of the red tape that goes with them. Taxes are a little trickier. They're compulsory, and most of us never even see the taxes we pay. Like the payments for many work-based health benefits, taxes are usually withheld—but not always. Millions of Americans (and illegal immigrants) don't pay taxes—so many that untaxed money transfers (income and sales) are estimated at $2 trillion per year, or about 15% of our economy. Some tax evaders are rich, and manage to hide millions, but over half are poor.*** Among the poor are most of the people who pay no income tax at all. They wouldn't pay much anyway, but they would be subject to withholding for social security, unemployment, and other entitlements. They avoid the tax, and forgo the benefits.

Most low-income American citizens don't pay taxes for two main reasons. The first is obvious: they don't want to. If someone who makes less that $25,000 per year receives that income under the table, why go on the tax rolls? The immediate effect of doing so would be reduction of nearly 10% in their take-home pay. Though there are some immediate benefits to filing, all involve forms, time and frustration, and they seldom match the withholding. How many working poor can afford that?

The second reason is less obvious: red tape. Most low-income tax evaders are not well-educated. To these working poor our tax code seems downright crazy. Maybe they've heard of the EZ 1040, but they hear a lot more about deductions, expenses, schedules, and accountants. They see their bosses struggle with these details, and they don't want to do it themselves. They assume that most tax headaches are caused more by complicated forms, requirements and rules than by the actual money. Many are driven more by the desire to escape the red tape than by the prospect of taxes themselves. They might be willing to enter a simpler, more straightforward tax system—one they could grasp quickly, whose benefits aren't mired in a bureaucratic maze. In the depths of the Depression many of the working poor accepted, and even welcomed, the introduction of payroll deductions for unemployment and social security. The taxes were simple, and in a time when most working Americans knew

---

*** http://taxvox.taxpolicycenter.org/2011/07/27/why-do-people-pay-no-federal-income-tax-2/ accessed on 2/14/12

firsthand about joblessness, and the poverty of their aging parents, they agreed to pay them. Would they have paid so cheerfully if they'd needed to pay a professional in the field just to figure how much they owed? No.

The same is true of healthcare. When a healthy, uninsured person commiserates with a friend undergoing medical treatments, the conversation is likely to turn to forms, regulations, coverage, and resources. For the seriously ill, red tape is a constant companion. Every new procedure brings reams of paperwork, and endless digital screens filled with requirements, warnings, and stipulations. When the patient isn't filling out something the doctor is. Real patients and actual medical procedures get lost in this storm of data. To the onlooker the paperwork often looks worse than the disease.

To an outside observer the process appears to be somewhere between tortuous and impossible. The idea that someone in his or her right mind would pay a monthly premium for such a thing could easily strike a healthy, uninsured person as nuts. Like anyone else, they dread the physical suffering that comes with disease, but they're terrified of the bureaucracy that goes with the cure.

The red tape starts wrapping around a sick person the moment he or she enters the system. In the ER there are forms to fill out. As soon as a healthcare practitioner sees the patient, the process escalates. Appearance, symptoms, diagnosis and prognosis all go into the records. The patient's chart grows. If specialists are brought in, the chart grows even faster.

Specialists tend to look at a case in terms of what's requested of them, and those requests usually revolve around their own fields. If I call in a cardiologist, the examination will begin with your heart. A neurologist will concentrate on your nervous system. They take other things into account, but they've been brought in to deal with a problem that's specific to their expertise.

At a hospital where I worked a 96-year old woman was brought in from a home for the elderly. The complaint that gained her admission was pneumonia. This woman was unaware of her surroundings, unresponsive, and dying. The instructions we had for her included a do-not-resuscitate (DNR) order. That's where our chart began. It shouldn't have even gotten that far. Ideally such a patient would remain in the home. She would be kept comfortable, and would be allowed to die. That's what's supposed to happen with DNR cases. But she was alive, and her children didn't want to put her on a respirator, so when she was diagnosed with pneumonia she wound up at our door.

During an examination a nurse found a drop of blood in the woman's diaper. This tiny spot wasn't sudden, surprising evidence that a healthy life was threatened. It couldn't be. This woman's healthy life was over, and she was near the end. The spot might have come from any one of multiple causes: a cut so small the nurse couldn't find it, or from the same kind of cut on the nurse's own hands. It might've gotten there when the diaper was being handled before it ever went on the woman. No one knew. The woman showed no other immediate warning signs, but now that she was in the hospital's care, this potential "problem" would be investigated and dealt with. This process began with the nurse reporting the blood spot to the internist/hospitalist in charge.

A hospitalist is a doctor who works exclusively in the hospital, with no outside practice. Like chameleons, some hospitalists take on the color of their surroundings, blending into the hospital environment, for good or for ill. A hospital survives on caution. A primary aim of all hospital policies is to avoid potentially litigious situations. For that reason policies are shaped to err on the side of caution. If we do everything, and then some, there's far less possibility of being successfully sued. Doctors who practice entirely within the hospital sometimes take this attitude to extremes.

In a perfect example of overzealous caution, when this hospitalist saw the blood spot, he called in the pertinent specialists for consultations. One came from a gynecologist and the other from a urologist. The gynecologist had a pap smear taken. That went into the woman's chart. The smear was analyzed, adding new data and pages to her record. That data led the gynecologist to call for more blood tests, and a pelvic sonogram. That way we would learn whether this dying woman had a life-threatening cancer, or other potentially dangerous conditions.

Meanwhile the urologist felt the spot required a urine test. This order went into the woman's record, and the next urine she produced was bottled, analyzed, and her chart got more lines and pages. If she had high urine sugar, or any one of several other complications, we would now know it. This reading material grew further when her doctors decided she needed a CAT scan.

I can't be sure about the nurse, but beyond her, the three doctors weren't really looking at the patient. Once the hospitalist learned about the drop of blood, his focus was on that, and whatever it might indicate. The gynecologist was concerned about problems in the reproductive system. The urologist was closely examining any difficulties in the woman's urinary tract. Their total billings certainly ran into the tens of thousands, if not more.

Why? Because three highly educated physicians, and various lab technicians and clerical workers, were using an array of costly equipment in a state-of-the-art medical facility to learn all there was to know about a drop of blood in a dying 96-year-old woman's diaper. Her real illness was pneumonia. A sick 96-year-old might be properly terrified of that, but she wasn't. She was unconscious. She was sick, but didn't know it, didn't care, and most likely would've just as soon died in peace. Instead she got numerous tests, generating a book-length chart before dying. Her treatment added nothing to her comfort. It wasn't a case for the annals of medical science, and added nothing essential to our knowledge. However, her chart added a great deal of documentation to justify bills that went out for pap smears, urine tests, and CAT scans. The bills were issued to insurance providers, Medicare, and possibly her family. That's how charts work. Each dose of a drug and each symptom add to the information. And every chart entry corresponds to records of price, coverage, and billing. That's how the hospital stays in business.

Today's doctor knows that her bill won't be based on what she's done. It will be based on what she can document. This documentation doesn't come from the unique situation of an individual patient, but from formulas based on measurable criteria that sometimes have little or nothing to do with the case. The doctor looks at whatever quantifiable data will fit her need for proper reimbursement. This isn't intentional fraud; it's the only way to get paid. The fraud is in a system that forces doctors to put bureaucracy's needs before those of the individual patient. Anyone who doubts this could find proof in the file cabinet of a family dentist. It's sparse. The dentist's records on a difficult patient who's had countless crowns, caps, root canals and fillings over several decades won't take up as much space as the hospital chart of a comatose pneumonia patient who arrived three days ago. Yet the dentist does the work, sends the invoice, and gets paid without much hassle. He's not a slave to his paperwork.

This documentation often bounces back at patients. More tests make more billing, and each bill increases the paperwork. Some insurers will lighten the patients' paperwork load, but there's no way to entirely eliminate it. This is the record of *your* health, so, if you change insurers, at the least you must make sure your records follow you. Every insured patient wants as little paperwork as possible. What sick person enjoys filling out more forms? When consumers shop around for health insurance, their questions often revolve around this issue. The savvy shopper asks: How complicated is it to get the insurer to pay? Will the healthcare provider invoice the insurer directly? Or do we get the bill, and, along with it, the responsibility of submitting it to our insurer? How do the co-payments work? Will we be billed for our portion separately? Or does this have to go through our insurance provider?

The answers to these, and other questions, vary from state-to-state, hospital-to-hospital, and insurer-to-insurer. One hospital visit can ensnare a patient in several different webs of bureaucracy, each with its own regulations. Many consumers are willing to pay higher premiums if a policy provides protection against this confusion. We realize that our insurer has charts on us too—huge piles of records that wind up in our files—and we want any records we deal with directly to be as brief and simple as possible. Consumers will give up money-saving deductibles and co-pay policies as long as their higher premiums guarantee freedom from bureaucratic snarls. It seems as if the only way for consumers to simplify their healthcare experience is to pay extra for it.

That should not be true.

In both taxes and health we now need an army of professionals simply to interpret the rules. Tax experts are usually either lawyers or accountants, with far more of the latter than the former. In health the experts go by several names, but the most prevalent is probably "patient advocate."

Over the last century accounting has grown up with the tax system. At first only businesses needed accountants, but with the dawn of the income tax came a bright new day for these professionals. As companies dealt with the ever-changing tax codes, their accounting departments grew, but accountancy's biggest boom was among individuals.

As Americans became more affluent, they paid higher tax rates. This brought pressure for the kind of loopholes and deductions businesses had always enjoyed. The sheer number of these breaks guaranteed complexity. That's when companies like H&R Block got big. We all wanted the complicated deductions, but we also dreaded that helpless feeling red tape inspires. Accountants knew how to make it all happen without any bother to us. We looked up from our boxes of unsorted schedules and receipts, and there stood a number cruncher who, for a few hundred bucks, could save us thousands, while reducing our role to that of signing the return. We brought them our piles of documents, which they accepted with a smile. We had no idea what they did, but we liked the results. They gave us time and saved us money. Who could argue with that?

Convoluted tax laws soon produced another powerful voice on the side of more complexity: the accountants themselves. Whenever legislators began to sound serious about tax simplification, the accounting lobby stopped them. Every deduction and loophole had its own special interest group, but accountants liked them all. These guaranteed their job security in an increasingly lucrative field. Today tens of millions of Americans use accountants, but we fear them too.

We praise them for curing our tax headaches, but we fear their ever-more-specialized knowledge of something so costly and incomprehensible.

In healthcare the patient advocate occupies a similar niche. Theirs is a relatively new profession, so it's not as pervasive—yet. Virtually nonexistent fifty years ago, in the last few decades patient advocacy has carved a place for itself as a necessary specialty. A good patient advocate can help financially-challenged patients wade through the thickets of bureaucracy, sometimes saving them substantial sums.

Back when medical care was limited, and relatively inexpensive, we got the bill, paid it, and that was that. But as therapies, treatments and medicines multiplied, many cases involved more and more providers and procedures. Costs often popped up piecemeal, and, as the field grew more complicated, patients faced an ever-growing array of choices. Often just one choice produced a confusing flurry of bills. It was enough to confuse anyone—even the insurers. While legislators and regulators insisted on giving patients full disclosure (which added more paperwork), manufacturers, providers, and insurers invented more and more things that had to be disclosed. Patients were soon lost in a blizzard of information that rivaled the tax labyrinth.

Patient advocacy got its earliest toeholds in hospitals, and that's where most of them still are. In the early days their primary job was simply to help the uninsured find the means to pay their bills. These advocates learned the ins and outs of government and nonprofit programs aimed at helping poor patients. In the 1960s Medicaid and Medicare were created to help the poor and elderly pay their medical bills. In those days the job was comparatively straightforward. Most of the time patients were treated, providers submitted their bills to the appropriate program, and eventually the bills were approved and paid. But over the years these programs added countless complications of their own. Innovations, errors and scandals were usually met with new regulations. When the new measures didn't cover every contingency, the standard solution was to add more.

Patient advocates now became experts at cobbling together packages from various resources. A patient's treatment often involves multiple personnel, drugs, procedures, and tools, each covered by a separate resource. One program might pay the internist, with another for the surgeon. A patient's insurance might fund the post-op check-ups, while a nonprofit pays for the meds. A veteran's program could cover a physical therapist, but when the patient needs a few days of home nursing, he or she might find that's not covered; then a supplementary policy might work. The advocate is supposed to know what's available, how to get it, and how to find resources to pay for it.

If we follow the logic of our present national health "policy," patient advocacy will grow like accounting did. This will occur with or without Obamacare. It will grow, as it does now, with increasing medical choices, and the accounting process will introduce an entirely new layer of complications. As treatment possibilities multiply, their finances will become more complex. Patient advocacy, private and public, will become as universally necessary in healthcare as CPAs are to taxes. In another decade most affluent Americans will meet with their personal patient advocates each year to review and adjust their coverage. The poor will be provided with this service through public health programs. (In many instances, this is already happening.)

But why should we go that route? Isn't the hands-on practice of modern medicine complex enough? With the plethora of treatment options, doctors and patients are already faced with many tough choices. The vast array of payment options adds another troubling layer of decision-making that often affects that patient's future wellbeing as much as the medical issues. Red tape causes stress, and stress can put a recovering patient right back in the sickbed. Supporters of patient advocacy contend that the profession is there to solve that problem, but many patients might see these advocates as one more layer of red tape. In many cases they're right. Often the patient advocate is just another person who's paid to make the system function, however haltingly. It's the standard bureaucratic fix: if the system doesn't work, add to it.

We can see this at work in a Maryland case several years ago when a teenaged bicyclist was hit by a car. The cyclist suffered a compound leg fracture, and some other less serious injuries. His mother was deceased, and his father was unemployed. His father arrived at the hospital just a few minutes after the ambulance, and, after seeing his son, immediately did his best to figure out how to pay for the boy's treatment. After successful surgery to set the bones, and an overnight stay, the boy was referred to a private facility for outpatient therapy.

The father emptied his bank account of $3,000 in savings, but that was all he had. The driver had only minimal insurance, which paid $10,000. It quickly became apparent that other bills would be at least $10,000 more (in the end the extra billings totaled $14,000), so the father approached one of the hospital's patient advocates. The advocate assured him that a Maryland state program would pay the rest, but later, when she filled out the forms, she didn't have the son's social security number. Instead of calling the father for this, she simply submitted the request without it.

Several weeks later the father received the program's denial of his claim. They didn't give a reason. He had no way of knowing what had really happened, so he assumed he simply hadn't qualified, and began looking for other resources. It wasn't until much later that he learned that the lack of a social security number was all that had stood between him and full payment of $14,000 in medical bills. If he'd learned of this within 90 days of the advocate's submission of the claim, he could've corrected it, but that deadline for resubmission had come and gone. The father had gotten another job, and he'd begun saving again, but a few months later the hospital took all it could from his account: $4,700. When he tried to get another of the hospital's patient advocates to help him he learned that they would no longer handle his case. It was now between the billing offices and him.

Much later, when it was all a bad memory, the father said: "There at the hospital you're traumatized. Your son's just arrived in an ambulance, doctors are operating on him, and you don't know what the hell is going on. Meanwhile, the staff guides you from desk to desk where people explain all this stuff. Each one gives you a logical, sympathetic explanation of something. You hardly know what, but you're grateful they're there to tell you. It seems like every explanation leads to a form. They've been telling you what it's for, so you sign it. The advocate is last. She tells you about a program that pays for everything. All you have to do is sign, and she will submit the forms to them. You leave her office feeling such relief. Then, over the next weeks and months, you lose everything."

Patients don't need to know every detail of medical finance any more than they need to be experts on medical science. It's not their job. Patients' jobs are to be aware of their own health, and to do all they can to stay healthy.

Doctors' jobs are to treat illness and injury, while helping their patients understand how complex medical issues affect them. It should be the job of institutions and insurers to set up systems whose costs and prices are not only transparent, but are also easy to understand. We don't need to create a whole new field of interpreters whose jobs depend on complication. We need to get into the habit of telling the simple truth.

Chapter Eight: The Wealth from Workers' Health

The red tape of healthcare isn't just a problem for patients; it plagues employers as well. For decades small business owners have been grappling with healthcare issues. Fifty years ago only a few small businesses offered their staff health benefits. That was starting to change, but the shift was gradual. It wasn't until the debates surrounding bills for Medicare and Medicaid that smaller businesses began looking seriously at the problem. In the next decade many employers made health insurance a standard benefit. Some who started covering their employees in the 1970s and early 1980s regretted the decision soon afterward. Medical advances and growing inefficiencies in the healthcare system caused insurance prices to skyrocket in the late '80s and early '90s, which led the Clinton administration to believe they could pass the nation's first comprehensive healthcare initiative. That failed, but in the mid-'90s the price increases abated somewhat, and popular support for a nationwide overhaul waned.

In the process many small business employers were left hanging. Fear of committing themselves to policies subject to steep future price hikes kept many of them from providing full coverage to employees, but legally they still had to insure them against health problems that were related to the job. Job-related injuries and illnesses were covered by workers' comp. For a business owner with just a few employees workers' comp could be relatively inexpensive, right up to the moment when someone filed a claim. If the employer chose to contest the claim, that took time and money. If the claim was approved, the price of the insurance went way up. Many small business owners avoided this in any way they could. It was a situation that pitted bosses against their own employees in businesses that relied on the two sides working in close proximity every day.

In 1997 the owner of a small boutique-style business in Annapolis, Maryland was wary of providing his shop manager with health coverage. With mostly part-time help, the manager was the business's only fulltime employee. When he began to get arthritis pains in his feet, ankles and knees, his medical bills quickly mounted. With pay of less than $25,000 per year, he soon went into debt, but when he talked to the owner about the possibility of getting health insurance, the owner was evasive. "If I insure you I'll be locked in," the man said. "When you leave the next guy will demand it, and I don't want to be committed to that."

When the manager related this to his doctor, the doctor said: "Your arthritis is job-related. You spend most of your day on your feet. It's not the total cause, but it's what's aggravating your joints. There are formulas for figuring out the percentages. That means you would qualify for workers comp. Just tell your boss I said that, and see what he does."

The manager told the owner, who immediately came around. Within a few days the owner instructed the manager to shop for a policy subject to the owner's approval. The manager found one that proved acceptable to both of them, and he had coverage within a month. From then on the policy paid the lion's share of his medical bills.

Why did the owner change his mind so quickly? The answer lay in the nature of workers' comp. If his manager filed for compensation, and the claim was accepted, this small business owner's workers' comp payments would go up, and stay up for several years—longer if any further claims were approved. If he fired the manager, that could easily raise issues concerning unemployment compensation, and create even more problems with workers' comp. Besides, the manager had been good at his job. In three years he'd helped boost the shop's sales considerably. If the owner fought the comp claim he knew it would create animus, and he would risk losing a valued employee. In either case, he would have paperwork coming out his ears—and, if he lost his manager, this was paperwork he would have to handle himself. In the end he knew that health coverage would be cheaper, less stressful, and he could get his happier, healthier manager to handle whatever paperwork it produced.

I've experienced this problem from a different perspective. Not all small business owners solve the problem in the same way, but most of them will go to some lengths to avoid workers' comp issues. They pay the premiums for the insurance because that's legally required, but when an employee has a work-related health issue, many bosses look for alternatives to this clogged, confused, and potentially money-draining system. An employee of a legitimate business, covered by workers' comp, will come into my office for treatment, and his boss will call, asking that we just send the bill directly to him. While he might be paying more in the short run, in the longer term he's keeping his workers' comp rates down, and avoiding potential conflicts concerning claims. In many cases this is the simplest, easiest and least expensive route.

Most workers' comp difficulties have their origins in a murky system that creates more problems than it solves. Workers' compensation is a thicket of rules, regulations, and laws, and all the potential conflicts that go with them. Over several decades the workers' comp system has created a body of law and court precedents so lengthy that large law firms have dedicated their entire workload to the specialty. These complications tempt any employer who has to deal with them to search for shortcuts. If the shortcut fails, most bosses either give in, or let the lawyers take over. With so many different players (workers, employers, insurers, doctors, regulators, arbitrators, and so on), all with narrow interests and different sets of rules, the system invites corruption.

Here in my home state of New York I've experienced one of the seamier examples of workers' comp in action. In New York we have a no-fault workers' comp system that's proved itself a recipe for shady dealings. As with any workers' comp system, it starts with employee claims of work-related conditions and disabilities. Workers who file disability claims need a diagnosis from a licensed doctor if they hope to have their claims approved.

Individual doctors tend to avoid this work for one simple reason: it doesn't pay much. The law caps the price, and, in the course of a normal medical practice, doing these diagnoses piecemeal isn't cost effective. The doctor might do it for a long-time patient, but many of these workers don't have a doctor they see regularly. Then there are the less-than-honest workers who don't trust their doctors to sign off on their claims. However, if you set up an office specializing in this, then do the most minimal examinations leading to the desired diagnoses, the heavy volume can produce plenty of profit. But this is dependent on holding down costs.

The owners of these medical offices keep their costs down in many ways: low-rent offices, outdated equipment, and low-paid medical staffers whose training and credentials often lack legitimacy. The staff will do brief examinations aimed at finding the malady. They make each diagnosis, documenting symptoms, and, whenever plausible, citing workplace causes. The most essential cog in this machine is the licensed physician. Every no-fault workers' comp office needs at least one. This doctor reviews the work, and signs off on the staff's findings.

In most of these offices, the legitimate doctor has the only job that pays a good salary. The only snag is in one's conscience. If a physician has any scruples, each paycheck comes with a corresponding loss of self-respect. Most of these licensed MDs are either near retirement, or desperate for work.

Years ago, when I was doing a job search, I answered an ad from one of these places. I'd heard some bad stories about them, but I assumed some must be on the level. Some probably are, but the one I visited was of the barely legal variety. My interviewers had some standard questions, but our conversation quickly came to the point: Could I produce a current license that I would allow them to affiliate with the address of the practice? If I could meet this one requirement, my job would consist of signing off on whatever their therapists said, giving their conclusions the necessary legitimacy. If I were to agree to be used this way they would hire me on the spot.

Of course I was suspicious, but I was also curious about how this place worked. Just how bad was it, I wondered. So I asked them, would I be expected to check the therapist's work? Well, of course I could, they said, but I should be aware that any changes to the therapist's conclusions would be discouraged. If I made a habit of altering the therapist's work, I could expect to be dismissed. After all, the therapist knew the score, so I should too. It was all just a matter of going along to get along. Though they weren't so crass to put it this way, they were operating under the assumption that their customers were always shopping for the most profitable diagnosis. The practice was in the business of providing it. After all, isn't the customer always right? No one ever said this out loud, but no matter how the language was disguised, this was how it worked.

Up to then I'd been warned about these places, but hearsay is never the same as seeing something up close. Now I knew from experience. The whole thing seemed surreal, so to check myself, I went over it with my wife. After listening to my account, and seeing the practice's pamphlet on work policies, she confirmed all my impressions. This place was every bit as compromised as I'd thought it was.

I turned down their lucrative offer, and abandoned any thought of trying a place like that again. Later I wasn't surprised to learn that many of these no-fault workers' comp offices had originally been semi-legitimate cash cows for the Mafia, the kind of business that could launder ill-gotten gains, while making a nice profit on its own. After a career in breaking legs and shooting rivals, a mobster would probably see this as a kinder, gentler investment—yet one where he could easily fit in. That gave me one more reason to be glad I'd turned down the job.

The idea of employers paying for work-related health problems is a good one. After all, these problems stem from workplace circumstances, and those are the employer's responsibility. But, like other sectors of healthcare and health insurance, workers' comp has grown into a huge maze of complexities. Lawyers, doctors, and insurers add new wrinkles to this all the time, and each new complication has its price. What's lost is any notion of justice, and what's left is whatever anyone can grab.

Chapter Nine: How Not to Learn about Medicine

There's medical information and medical misinformation, and they often overlap. The patient is the beginning of that information. The patient's body is the source of his or her medical needs and knowledge. In the ideal world of Marcus Welby, or even ER, a good patient pays attention to what he or she feels. This patient learns to report these feelings to the physician —especially changes, pains, and deteriorations—with as much accuracy as possible. The patient doesn't need to know any medical terminology. Clear everyday language will do. If the patient can convey location, intensity, duration, and other specific qualities of a feeling, a competent doctor will know the technical terms.

The good doctor listens closely to the patient, and examines both the whole, and the particular. The best doctors are more than competent at reading data from machines and tests, but they also never lose track of the fact that the patient is what counts. What's right there in front of the doctor's eyes? How does this patient look and feel, and how does that stack up against tests and history? The doctor assembles a whole picture, giving context to the individual ailment. He or she then prescribes treatments, therapies and/or drugs, and monitors results. Until the problem is solved or controlled, the doctor continues to listen to the patient's report. Even when the ailment is cured, the doctor recalls this process in any further treatment of the patient.

This is the ideal. Most of us know that we seldom reach an ideal, but it does give us a clear yardstick by which we measure real life behaviors. The comparison tells us whether we're doing better or worse. The key to achieving anything resembling this ideal situation is communication. The patient relates symptoms as precisely as possible, and answers the doctor's questions. The doctor listens, and strives to make his or her questions and recommendations clear.

This doesn't mean the patient has to rely solely on the physician for data. A savvy patient will ask the doctor about reading material, websites, and other sources. A smart, curious patient won't be expected to stop there. If the patient finds other information that veers toward different conclusions, he or she should not be afraid to bring this up. But a patient should also have enough trust in his or her doctor to listen to any diagnosis and prognosis, and to grant the doctor the authority necessary for successful treatment. That's real communication. It's a two-way street.

Direct-to-consumer advertising in print and electronic media is not communication; it's nothing more than the old-fashioned Madison Avenue sales pitch. There's a difference. When a doctor and patient converse about the patient's health, both have special knowledge of unique subject matter: that patient's body. The patient knows it from the inside, and the doctor knows it from informed observation and training. Their discussions are anchored in the same context, and they are looking at the same problem. They convey information in a dynamic process, allowing for give-and-take. That can't happen in a mass market ad campaign.

An advertisement is a one-way street running directly at you. An ad beaming out through mass media is automatically aimed at as wide an audience as possible—a million yous. Though advertisers routinely target a product's primary audience, advertising is, by its nature, welcoming, inclusive, and bent on attracting all the positive attention it can. Take an ad for a prescription drug to relieve the pains of arthritis. This ad will be aimed at those who are middle-aged and older. It begins with the image of the gimpy 50-year-old father rubbing his aching legs, then dissolves into one of him giving the new bottle of pills a hopeful look. With optimistic dialogue and narration, the scene shifts to the man shooting baskets with his teenaged son. Obviously the ad is aimed at viewers as old, or older than the onscreen father. However, it's also designed to nudge younger family members into thinking of the drug as a great solution for dear old dad's aches and pains. The ad makers know that if they broaden their target to include the whole family, spouses and children will talk about the drug with the advertisers' prime target: the middle-aged arthritic patient. They design the ad to defy its inherent limitations, and cast as a wide net as possible.

But limitation is the main goal of the prescription process. The idea behind prescription requirements is to direct potentially harmful drugs only to those patients who need them for their beneficial effects. Quantity, refills, and dosages are all limited, and this is documented, usually right on the bottle. All of these precautions are created to deal with potential danger. Often the danger is simply in the newness of the drug. It's been tested on animals and humans, but there are still reasonable questions about its potential problems. These might not show up until a larger population has used it for longer periods. Over time the drug develops a history, and if it proves both benign and beneficial, the FDA can approve it for over-the-counter sales. That's happened with countless drugs, from pain relievers to allergy medications.

Some drugs remain restricted because the only way to protect patients from their dangers is through close monitoring. As I've noted elsewhere, when penicillin came on the market in the late 1940s it changed history. Countless lives were saved, infections were stopped in their tracks, and formerly dangerous surgeries became routine. But penicillin could hurt, or even kill an allergic patient.

Over time researchers developed other antibiotics. The first of these served as substitutes for penicillin, giving allergic patients the same benefits. As more and more were concocted, scientists became familiar with their properties, and began designing antibiotics targeted toward increasingly specialized purposes. One might work best on skin problems. Another would work only in the intestines. Some were used in animal feed, while others were deemed safe enough to go into over-the-counter products. Some of the new antibiotics had the possibility of dangerous side effects. To this day penicillin and most of its cousins can only be bought with a prescription. Many of us have had, or know people who've had, allergic reactions to antibiotics. This class of wonder drugs has gained a schizophrenic reputation, making them less attractive subjects for advertising. Some patients ask for them, but others are leery. Periodically we see waves of news stories about claims that physicians prescribe these miraculous antibiotics far too much. Many of the stories are true. Whenever a doctor prescribes penicillin for a cold, the patient should ask why. The drug won't do anything to the cold. Perhaps this is why we don't see that many prescription antibiotics being promoted on TV. But they are becoming the exception.

Then there's the world of negative interactions with other drugs. As we develop more and more pharmaceuticals that do more and more things, inevitably some will not go well with others. An ad concentrates on a single drug, and its stated purpose. The ad will look at the patient who benefits, and has no complications. That way we can clearly see what the drug is supposed to do. Advertisers design the disclaimers to have as little effect as possible, pitting a low, hurried voice against a series of happy images. They don't belabor the negative. After all, they want us to buy the product. That's their job.

Direct-to-consumer (DTC) advertising is a recent phenomenon. Up until the 1970s there were virtually no DTC ads for doctors, lawyers, or prescription drugs. In 1977 that started to change when two Arizona lawyers appeared before the Supreme Court arguing against their recent suspension from that state's bar association. The Arizona Bar had suspended them for advertising their firm on TV. The lawyers had run ads for a practice specializing in helping people of moderate income to secure government grants. It was an area where the only way to make real profits was to produce a high volume of cases. These two lawyers decided that running DTC ads was the only way to attract enough business.

Before the Court they argued that they were entitled to run the ads under the free speech provision in the First Amendment. In keeping with traditions that went back to the beginning of the 20th century (when mass media was just being born), the Arizona Bar Association opposed them. The Court agreed with the lawyers' basic arguments on free speech, but also allowed the Bar Association to regulate ads somewhat. It seemed like a nuanced decision, but its real effect was to open the floodgates. Soon lawyers were advertising in almost every medium: print, TV, radio, and more recently, the Internet.

By the early 1980s pharmaceutical companies were getting into the act. As with lawyers, their first forays into DTC were timid tests of the system. These early attempts revealed an increasingly lenient attitude on the part of regulators and legislators.

Another factor that pushed pharmaceutical manufacturers to increase their DTC advertising was a decrease in their ability to market directly to doctors. For many years pharmaceutical sales forces had treated physicians to lunches, dinners, golf outings, and even vacations in ritzy resorts. They often aimed at the youngest doctors—medical residents and interns working in hospitals. These were the ones working high-pressure, low pay, entry-level jobs. Enduring hundred-hour work weeks filled with endless crises, these new physicians were ready for anyone who could give them a restful break. Sales reps knew that if they could establish a positive relationship with a doctor who was just starting out, they could push new pills to his patients for decades thereafter. With their growing cornucopia of wonder drugs, and their enticing meals and junkets, these marketers could command the attention of almost any young doctor.

By the early '90s hospital directors took notice. They knew the influence a good salesman could have on a young, exhausted mind. Pharmaceutical direct-to-doctor sales methods were beginning to draw negative media attention. While the drug industry's sales forces were still offering anything that was legal, the hospital directors began placing their own limits on what their staff doctors could accept. Many of the most attractive sales methods were forbidden. There were less free vacations, less golf games, and less lunches. If the party wasn't over, it was at least toned down.

With these traditional sales venues choked off, drug sellers had to find new ways to get patients interested. Up to now they'd relied on the authoritative voice of the doctor. There in the office, patients listened, and most did exactly what their physicians told them to do. That would still be true, but as institutions threw up barriers around their staff doctors, drug salesmen had to find new ways to influence those physician-patient conversations. The simplest solution was to appeal directly to the people who would pop the pills:

the patients themselves. If they went to their doctors demanding the newest prescription drugs—drugs that would be protected for years by patents—the doctors would surely give them what they wanted.

Drug manufacturers adopted this strategy just as baby boomers were reaching middle age. Over 78 million Americans were born between 1946 and 1964—the largest generation in our history. The boomers had grown up with new drugs, both legal and illegal. Unlike earlier generations, they weren't that afraid of self-medication. They and their friends were likely to have experienced everything from aspirin to LSD. Boomer patients and their children easily accepted this new notion of going into one's doctor to demand a specific medication. This dovetailed perfectly with the drug sellers' emerging marketing strategy. The TV ads increased.

By the late 1990s viewers, listeners and readers were all being inundated by ads for prescription drugs. The sensational new erectile dysfunction drug, Viagra, led the way. How could anyone resist a drug that virtually guaranteed better sex? These new and effective sex enhancers were tailor-made for creative ad men. Finally they could come right out and say to America: "Sex is healthy. We all want it. Now your doctor can help you get it whenever you want." It was Madison Avenue's dream come true. They'd always used sex to sell other products. Now sex itself was the product, and they could market it directly to the buyer. How could they miss?

DTC physician advertising followed a similar path. In the 1970s Marcus Welby would've had his license suspended if he'd run ads on TV—much like the Arizona lawyers. Of course, the good Dr. Welby never even considered it. He would soon be behind the times. Within a couple of decades hospitals, clinics, and physician practices were advertising tummy tucks, joint replacement, and cancer treatments.

Now we're used to watching an ad for a prescription drug, then another for a doctor who'll prescribe it. We go to the doctor, demand the prescription, then stop at our local pharmacy to get it filled. Six months later, when the drug has produced every downside its long disclaimer promised, resulting in that final side effect: death, our heirs call the number in an ad for a malpractice lawyer. When she wins their claim, they give her a video testimonial for her next ad. What a vicious cycle!

So how did Dr. Welby manage without these modern advantages? Lacking this free flow of information, how could patients possibly know what doctor to go to, or what drugs they might want? And if the patient doesn't know what he or she wants, how's the poor doctor going to know what prescription to write?

Marcus Welby didn't wait to be told what the patient wanted. He felt his job was to do whatever the patient *needed*. What the patient wanted was a given in those days: the patient's strongest desire was to know what was wrong, and how to fix it. They wanted to get well. In those days the doctor was the one who was supposed to know how to make them whole again. Welby listened, watched, examined, and diagnosed the problem. He then put it in plain English for the patient. If it was a complex ailment requiring highly technical treatment, he did his best to help his patient understand what was happening. All the while he paid strict attention to his patient's concerns and reactions. They communicated.

Back then the closest Dr. Welby came to advertising was a couple of lines of block print in the local yellow pages. Lawyers—even ambulance chasers—were confined to roughly the same thing. In those days the only pharmaceutical ads were in medical trade journals. Drug companies targeted the doctors themselves, with ads steeped in technical information only doctors would understand. The doctors were expected to translate all this jargon into language the patient could comprehend.

As we've seen, the companies marketed aggressively, but laws, regulations, and traditions kept a tight rein on DTC drug promotion. As a whole, society regarded the idea of medical and legal DTC ads in a negative light. Patients and potential litigants didn't demand a change. Drug makers, physicians and lawyers did. Like any active participants in a capitalistic society, these service providers wanted to attract new business any way they could.

***

Today many patients walk into their doctors' offices with lengthy lists of therapies and prescriptions. They've seen the drugs on TV, and they want them. Some doctors try to dissuade patients, while others look for any excuse to give in to their demands. Like any other service providers, some doctors concern themselves with honest high-quality work, while others are more comfortable with a high volume practice aimed at each customer's immediate gratification.

For a conscientious doctor these are everyday headaches. We're trained to observe, test, diagnose, and prescribe the proper course of action, but increasingly we are faced with patients who have their own ideas about what we should be giving them. The 50-year-old man wants the pill that can help him shoot baskets, and next week his wife comes in wanting the pill she saw on the Internet that promises to give her the energy of youth.

Recently a patient we will call "Lisa B" arrived in our offices. This 28-year-old mother of two, with a new baby at home, had been complaining to her obstetrician about her symptoms of post partum depression. He'd referred her to her primary physician who'd started her on Prozac two months earlier. So far Lisa hadn't been able to get in for a follow-up, but when her depression persisted, she started paying more and more attention to the advice she got from the TV screen.

There she saw an ad for Abilify. She'd heard about this drug from a girlfriend who also had depression. The girlfriend had told Lisa that her doctor had prescribed Abilify to go with her other meds. The girlfriend had been quite happy with the effects of the combination.

The TV ad seemed aimed directly at Lisa. It followed a woman of about her age, while a soft-voiced narrator told viewers that anti-depressants don't always do the whole job. Women like Lisa might need something more to augment their primary medication. Naturally, the announcer suggested that Abilify would do the job. As is usually the case with drugs aimed at depression, the ad's approach was subtle. No shots of laughter here—just the woman, eyes brightening and gradually becoming more alert as the ad went on. There she was, talking to a co-worker, then going to a movie with a friend. The standard litany of suicide warnings and death threats played out against a walk on a dock with seagulls swaying on the breeze. Now the telegenic young woman smiled sweetly, and spoke up for the drug. With a confident air she simply said: "Adding Abilify has made a difference for me." It was a study in the art of the soft sell. The ad did its job, pushing Lisa directly into our office. She wanted Abilify.

While describing her symptoms, Lisa was frank about her history of depression and bipolar disorder. She also had asthma, and there was the birth of her second child four months earlier. Her thoroughness about these things was impressive. From that it would be easy to assume she was telling us everything. When we asked her for a complete list of her medications, she told of the daily Prozac, Xanax as needed, and she used an asthma inhaler. Lisa reported no side effects from any of these. She was free of hallucinations, and hadn't been subject to homicidal or suicidal thoughts. Still the Prozac-Xanax regimen had left her with some anxiety and depression just about every day. She wanted those symptoms to go away.

Our physical exam showed nothing extraordinary. Lisa seemed like a nice woman with normal vital signs, and no obvious distress. In her psychiatric exam, she demonstrated a mildly depressed mood, but nothing beyond what she had described on arrival. We saw no concerns with her speech, attention, thought or judgment. These were about what one would expect from a young woman who has mild but persistent depression. We discussed possible treatments with her, including counseling and stress reduction management techniques. We also explored her family situation. There didn't seem to be any family problems, but she didn't want to bother them with something that could be solved with a pill. Like many of today's patients, she saw drugs as the primary solution to most psychiatric disorders.

Her post partum depression (a condition that often shows up briefly after childbirth) had lasted longer than usual. This wasn't that surprising. Lisa's family history included depression, and I knew she'd received medications that were markers of earlier depressive issues. If she hadn't seemed frank, and hadn't asked for anything specific, I would've referred her to a psychiatrist for immediate assessment and treatment. But Lisa knew what she wanted, and she had her reasons. She'd been impressed by her friend's experience, so when the commercial came on she was already prepped to be swayed by it. She wanted to completely banish her depression, and now she thought she knew how. I was simply the one who had the proper credentials to help her do it.

I was willing to do that, as long as she also agreed get her regular doctor to recommend a psychiatrist. That way her regular doctor would be onboard, and the psychiatrist would help her see how all this fit in with her overall condition. Lisa's only problem was a faulty memory. When she'd listed the prescription drugs she'd been taking she'd forgotten one. If I'd known of it, I never would've prescribed anything stronger than Tylenol.

A week later Lisa's husband brought her back to us. She was in distress. Her eyes were physically locked into an upward gaze, and she was running a fever of 102°. This condition had shown up early that morning. At first she'd hoped it would go away, but when it didn't her husband insisted that she come in.

We recognized her condition as an Oculogyric Crisis, which is a form of Tardive Dyskinesia (TD). It's a well known and not terribly uncommon condition that Abilify can exacerbate. In the course of the visit her husband revealed that Lisa had been prescribed Oxycodone (Percocet) after the delivery of her second child. She'd forgotten to include that in her list of medications. It was an important omission. Together these drugs can cause Neuroleptic Malignant Syndrome, or NMS, which can be fatal. Once we saw this danger, we got Lisa to a hospital. There they found that she did have a full-blown case of NMS, and they put her in the ICU. She was there for two weeks. NMS doesn't end with a hospital stay, and Lisa returned home to a long period of recovery.

Then there was Jeanine W, a 36-year-old in reasonably good health. When Jeanine arrived at an obstetrician's office, she and her husband already had three children, and they did not want more. Jeanine had been using various methods of contraception, but felt she needed a break from them. Options such as a vasectomy for her husband, or her own sterilization, were not acceptable to the couple. (She was reporting this; her husband wasn't with her.) She and the OB discussed various options, but Jeanine had seen ads for YAZ birth control on TV. The OB discussed the risks with her, but she was adamant. Jeanine didn't smoke, or have high blood pressure or a family history of stroke. The doctor didn't see anything in her history that would predict complications, so he agreed, giving her a prescription for YAZ.

Five months later Jeanine suffered a debilitating stroke. The neurologist on her case named YAZ as the probable culprit. Now a mother of three will have to relearn basic life skills. It's likely that she will need assistance for the rest of her life.

***

There have always been some doctors who would prescribe just about anything a patient asked for, but most of us have seen them as quacks. In the past most patients regarded doctors who were too quick with their prescription pads as something less than reputable. If we trusted our doctor, we assumed he or she would know the best prescription, even if it didn't precisely fit our own ideas.

DTC has changed that. A patient who comes in demanding a specific drug wants a willing doctor. Getting the drug conditions a patient to see this as a normal course of action in today's medical care. We monitor our bodies, watch the TV ads, and decide what we want. We see our MDs in much the same way our parents looked at their pharmacists, regarding a physician's expertise as a mere adjunct to the media's authority. We allow the media to be our primary medical advisor. When we hear information coming from a radio, or see it on a screen, or read about it in print, we pay attention. The ad advises us to ask to our doctor about it.

That would make sense if they wanted us to go to our doctors with intelligent questions about a drug, but that's not how it works, and the ad makers know it. When they tell us to ask our doctor about it, many patients ask only one question: Will you give me the drug?

Too many doctors have the experience of saying no, then never seeing that patient again. We might have a doctor who's firm with his patients, criticizing doctors who act like pill salesmen. A longtime patient comes in demanding the latest feel-good drug, and the doctor says no. The patient politely tells him their relationship is over, and walks out the door. After such an experience, the doctor might say no again, but the next time his voice quavers. The patient walks out, and the doctor knows he's seen that one for the last time. Finally, fearing the loss of even more patients, he caves in. After all, other doctors are doing it, aren't they? He gives the next patient the requested drug. The doctor justifies this by telling himself that the patient will be better off if a concerned physician is actually monitoring the case. He's sorry he couldn't do that for the earlier patients who left him. And he no longer carps about doctors who give in to every patient demand.

Medicine's old phrase for this was "satisfaction of search." In earlier times that might have meant finding a good doctor who could make a positive difference in one's health. Today it's finding a doctor who'll do what you want done, much like "customer satisfaction" at the retail level.

This brings in a silent undercurrent of "the customer is always right," increasing the pressure on doctors to grant every wish. We go in for a cold, demanding an antibiotic. We have a pain, so we simply must have a painkiller. I want a sexual stimulant, while you feel you need the latest medication for acne. We used to talk to our pharmacist about over-the-counter fixes. Now we go to our doctor's office, wanting the more restricted stuff. At one time that wouldn't have occurred to most patients, but DTC has changed that. Now the ads urge us to go see our doctor. The wording is careful, but the message is not. They tell us to ask our doctors about it, but what we're supposed to hear is: Go ask your doctor for this drug. After all, isn't that what he's there for?

***

Lawyers—so many of whom build their livelihoods on DTC ads—will argue that DTC advertising is a simple First Amendment issue. They say the Bill of Rights guarantees freedom of speech and freedom of the press, two of the main bulwarks of our overall freedom of thought and expression. But that's a narrow view. Though a lawyer might prove his point by citing court decisions and precedents, there is another way to look at it.

Like any real communication tool, freedom of speech is a two-way street. It's not just our right to proclaim our ideas out loud. It's also our right to have access to all the information we need for life, liberty and the pursuit of happiness. We're free to say what we want, and, just as important, we're free to hear whatever's out there. These rights have a purpose: a society of informed individuals. The theory is that the more we can learn, the better chance we have of understanding the truth. If the theory works, the truth will make us free.

Medicine is the art and science of healing and keeping the body healthy. If we're to enjoy life and liberty, while pursuing our happiness, good health is our most basic tool. That means we need the facts about drugs and doctors. We should know the good and the bad. We want a balanced view of benefits and drawbacks, but that goes against the core purpose of advertising. Advertising is the art of selling. Though dishonesty isn't always inherent in advertising, the line between true and false easily blurs, especially when the ad deals with a product's negative factors. Ads aren't meant to scare us away, or even to caution us. Their aim is to tell us all that's good about a product, while downplaying any difficulties. Drug ads put this principle on display. Every image is positive. The people taking the drug are healthy, happy and smiling.

The positive principle is most evident in the one negative part of the commercial: the disclaimer. We've heard about the miracles this drug can bring, and we've seen the 50-year-old arthritis patient go from gimpy old man to athlete in a little less than a minute. Fueled by the new pain reliever, he keeps shooting baskets with his teen-aged son, while a low-pitched, fast-talking monotone runs through a laundry list of symptoms long enough to sedate an amphetamine addict. In another ad, this one for an ED drug, a smiling couple shares warm, lecherous leers in their hot tub, while the same monotone warns against the four-hour erection. These disclaimers get the precise reactions the advertisers are aiming for: mild chuckles the first time, and then deafness every time after. That's how a good ad deals with bad data: by being thorough, boring, dismissive, and subtly comic.

An excellent argument could be made that DTC advertising in medicine inhibits free speech. Patients watching these ads are being conditioned to see only one side of the issue. The treatment of the disclaimer is bound to carry over to the patient's use (or lack of use) of the insert information that comes with the drug. All the patient wants to know is whether the pain will go away, or whether tonight's the night he'll get lucky. Once the patient has asked for the prescription, bought the drug, and opened the bottle, his only concern is whether the pill works. If it does, he won't care about disclaimers. If he suffers that threatened bout of priapism, he can turn on the TV, and find a lawyer who specializes in cases like his. Just call this number, and...

Chapter Ten: Taking Care of Business

When a problem affects all of society, one of the first places we look for solutions is education. We always wonder: Can better schooling help? When the modern Civil Rights movement got started after World War II the first issue to gain traction was the integration of schools. We assumed that if children were educated together they would learn to live together. When Russia beat us into space with the first tiny satellite, America turned to its teachers, who redoubled their efforts to train our children in math and science. Whenever matters of faith become public policy issues, the role of public and private education is always high on the agenda. Whether it's saying no to drugs, or stopping bullying, we like to begin our efforts in the classroom. It's the one place where everyone is supposed to listen.

So what about healthcare?

In the last half-century few issues have been debated with more passion. Few problems have taken up more of our time. Nothing—not even defense—has cost more. In the '60s we argued over Medicare and Medicaid, in the '70s malpractice took center stage, the '80s were a time of rising insurance costs, followed by the failed Clinton healthcare bill in the '90s. More recently we've been dealing with Obamacare, and there's still no end in sight. Yet, in fifty years of intense debate, medical education has always been a side issue. There's never been much national discussion about how medical schools deal with the business, ethics, or personal finance issues that define so much of the doctor/patient relationship.

What would a patient expect to find in his or her doctor's education? That's easy. Aside from the technical and scientific aspects of medicine, a medical school might be expected to teach a thorough course in medical ethics. What's right? What's wrong? Why? And how does a doctor work through ethical questions to reach the most ethical answers? This affects every aspect of what a doctor does.

Next a patient might expect a doctor to have some rudimentary understanding of the basic principles of business. It's not that every doctor needs a keen business sense, but every doctor is in a business, and we should know the basics. We perform services, use materials, and run practices, clinics, hospitals, and other healthcare facilities. We require payment from our patients, and we must pay our own bills. We have to make sure there's more money coming in than going out. We have corporations, partnerships, sole proprietorships and nonprofits. We deal with everything from stock options to payroll taxes. We're all a part of a $3 trillion-per-year industry. By most measures it's the largest sector of our economy. If that's not a business, what is?

A patient also has every right to expect a doctor to have some understanding, and to take an interest in how personal finance affects the patient's choices. When a doctor sets out a course of treatment with no thought to the patient's ability to pay, it can seem like tantalizing torture. The patient becomes the proverbial kid peering through the candy store window—all those goodies just a few feet away, behind an insurmountable barrier.

But we're not talking about treats here. Healthcare is a life-giving necessity that's also one of the largest items in any normal household budget. Anyone who has health insurance knows this. Insurance premiums are the biggest cost, and if someone gets sick, additional deductibles, co-pays, and procedures not covered by the policy, can mount up into the tens of thousands. Most healthcare-based bankruptcies happen to people who are insured. If a sick patient sees treatment as a looming financial meltdown, it's bound to affect his or her mental state, influencing the medical outcome. A doctor who ignores this is neglecting an essential component in the patient's health.

Too often a patient goes to a new doctor, and as the two of them go over the patient's health issues, the doctor recommends treatments. The doctor might ask some general question about the patient's ability to pay, and often he or she will ask if the patient's insurance has any drug coverage. But doctors seldom ask for any details about this. It's easier to regard money matters as the patient's personal business, and not a fit subject for probing.

This often leads to a doctor recommending treatments and prescribing drugs that the patient can't afford. The doctor might give the patient a free sample of the latest drug for high blood pressure. The patient goes through the sample, her blood pressure goes down, and the doctor writes her a prescription. It's only when she gets to the drugstore that she realizes her annual co-pay on this medicine will be in the thousands—an amount she simply can't afford. Had the doctor known, he could've prescribed an older, cheaper drug. As it is, there's a good possibility that this patient will never return to this doctor. Her experience tells her she can't afford what he's offering. She may find this embarrassing, or she might simply regard the doctor's approach as unrealistic.

It would make more sense for a doctor to have a reasonably good notion of a patient's ability to pay. This might seem like an imposition that borders on an invasion of privacy. It's not. Think of it in terms of two other businesses that take up a lot of our time and money: homes and cars.

When we want to buy a home we go to a realtor. The realtor asks us what we can afford, and often asks permission to check our credit rating. A smart realtor won't show a client a house that's not in the client's price range. She knows it's a waste of time.

Once we find a house we like, we go to the bank. The bank's loan officer wants a detailed picture of our finances: salary, assets, debts, and any other potential obligations. Even during the real estate boom, when some banks were lending money to anyone with an active pulse, bankers still asked these questions. When it turned out that they weren't paying attention to the answers, or were falsifying them, the public saw it as an industry-wide scandal. Now that the boom has turned to bust, the bankers are paying attention again. The realtor can't afford to have a client sign a contract that won't be honored. The bank can't afford any more bad loans on its books. This is business at its most basic. They only sell to those who can pay.

We go through a similar process when buying a new car. The car dealer looks at our credit score and history. She asks questions about our jobs, incomes, and financial obligations. The dealer wants to be sure we'll come up with the monthly payment. If we can't satisfy her requirements, she won't sell us the car. Though ultimately a sick patient must get the proper healthcare, whether he pays or not, he will be responsible for finding financial resources. Why shouldn't a doctor's office or hospital take as much interest in a patient's financial condition as a car dealer does?

Most of us think of our houses and cars as the most costly items we will ever buy. A lot of us will spend thirty years making our monthly mortgage payments. Over that time we'll buy several cars, adding more to our monthly expenses. Before we're allowed to take on these debts we'll be questioned, scrutinized, and judged. That's not the case when we enter a healthcare facility.

In a hospital, clinic, or doctor's office the only thing we're sure to be asked about is our insurance. If we don't have any, and the medical problem is potentially expensive, but not an acute emergency, we'll probably be referred elsewhere. Many uninsured have gone through this. When the patient calls Dr. A's office the receptionist asks, and learns that there's no insurance. The receptionist refers the patient to Dr. B. Dr. B's receptionist asks the same question, gets the same answer, and gently suggests that the patient call Dr. C, whose office routinely refers such cases to Dr. D. Dr. D's standard uninsured referral might be to Dr. A, starting the process over again. If the patient is lucky, he's gotten well by now. If not, he'll keep looking until his condition worsens, gaining emergency status. Then he'll call the ambulance.

The oddity is that, while most such patients are working poor, it's not their income or assets that determine their fate. An uninsured patient with a million-dollar bank account might go through the same round-robin. If he brings up his net worth, the receptionist in the doctor's office often won't know how to process that information. She doesn't have any formulas for assets-to-treatment costs. None of her bosses have mentioned anything about patients' assets or bank balances. Few medical offices do credit checks. Insurance is the Holy Grail.

In most cases a patient doesn't even need insurance that covers her problem. Her policy might have a huge deductible, or require large co-pays that could soar into the tens of thousands. If the patient has a serious malady, past due bills might bankrupt her before her insurance pays a dime. But if the patient produces a bona fide insurance card most medical facilities will admit her with little or no further scrutiny. A bank's loan officer would be appalled. A realtor's jaw would drop. A car dealer would examine the process carefully, asking: "How does this racket work?"

This isn't to say that patients without means should be turned away. The point of these observations is that our entire medical system is so disjointed that it often seems the normal rules don't apply. Everyone's in it for the profit, yet medicine isn't supposed to be about making money. Everyone's in it to heal wounds and cure disease, but they also need to make a reasonable living. Individuals need paychecks, companies need profits, and research needs funding. But why does all this cost so much more here in the U.S. than it does in other countries?

Does supply fit demand? No one knows. Do prices reflect costs? Not at all. Doctors, insurers, hospitals, drug and equipment manufacturers—none of them really know how the business of medicine works. They only know how their narrow part of it functions. A doctor probably knows how her practice keeps afloat, with patients coming in, bills going out, and the various monthly expenses being paid. The insurer knows averages and percentages: how many policyholders are likely to be well, how many are likely to be sick, and how sick they're likely to be. Insurers know what doctors and hospitals will charge. Often they dictate these charges. Hospital administrators know averages and percentages too, but from a different perspective. They keep up on the most effective billing and payment strategies, which change all the time. They execute those strategies in an atmosphere that's surreal at best.

Medical education doesn't address this. Aspiring doctors learn healing skills, but they don't learn business practices. We might take the Hippocratic Oath, but we aren't required to take courses covering medical ethics. We want to do all we can to heal our patients, but nothing in our education encourages us to pay attention to their financial situations.

Some people in medicine recognize the problem, and want to face it head on. More and more medical schools are offering joint M.D./M.B.A programs, 65 at last count.[*] However these are optional, and many of the medical students who complete these programs soon wind up in healthcare administration or finance. Once that happens they're no longer in the business of seeing patients.

Not every doctor needs an M.B.A, but all doctors should have some business training. On one internet site Jay Agarwal writes: "An effective and very feasible solution to educating future physicians with the business skills they need to inspire their entrepreneurial minds would be to incorporate a compact and basic business course throughout the first few years of medical school."[**]

The course could include training in patient finance. The doctor wouldn't have to ask all the questions. Most of that could be done by staff when the patient first comes in. Patients already fill out forms, and those could be adapted to elicit the pertinent data. What's the patient's income? Does he own a car? A home? Staffers could be authorized to check credit scores. Insurance cards could be modified to show deductibles and co-pay formulas. Staffers could then give the doctor the most essential information about the patient's ability to pay. The doctor doesn't need to know every detail. The data could be combined into something like a traditional credit rating. Formulas would be standardized, and scores would be private, but the smart patient would authorize the

---

[*] "Adjusting, More M.D.'s, Add M.B.A." by Milt Freudenheim, *New York Times,* September 5, 2011, accessed 4/11/12

[**] "A place for business in medical school" by Jay Agarwal, http://www.kevinmd.com/blog/2011/09/place-business-medical-school.html, accessed 4/11/12

facility to access them. There could be a score to show the quality of the patient's insurance coverage for treatments and therapies, another for drug coverage, and finally a score for his or her overall financial status. The doctor would consider these scores when prescribing drugs and recommending treatments.

A medical student's education in business and finance would be connected to schooling in ethics. Medical ethics and the Hippocratic Oath would be augmented by business ethics. Students would study the ethical problems that arise when treating financially-challenged patients. When is it appropriate to substitute a cheaper drug? What ethical criteria does a doctor use when devising an effective treatment program that's within the patient's means?

If these matters were adequately explored in medical school doctors and other healthcare professionals might find themselves looking at other issues in a different light. How would this approach affect a physician's ideas about TV ads? With proper training in patient finances and business ethics, would doctors give out drug samples the same way they do now? Most doctors would learn to be more sensitive to their patients' ability to pay.

Changes in education almost always bring about unexpected results. What's taught in school gets tested and tempered when students bring it into the real world. But if the medical community were to take these things seriously we could bring a far more sensible logic to everything we do. We could rededicate the medical profession to a more realistic, more effective approach to what we do best: healing injuries and curing diseases.

Chapter Eleven: Patient Responsibility: Let the Buyer Beware

So far we've concentrated on the medical profession and insurers: the supply end in the healthcare market. But what about the consumer? Healthcare is a transaction between the provider and the patient. Insurers, and any other sources of funds, are third parties, whose direct involvement only comes later, when bills are due. An insurer has an obligation to pay any bills covered by the patient's policy. A doctor is required to address the patient's maladies, and recommend treatments. But what are the patient's obligations? In a word, they are: *huge*.

Your body isn't just something you own, it's something you *are*. As long as you are conscious, sane and able to control your movements, you are the first responder to your needs. You are the one with the heartbeat, you own the brain waves, you have the metabolism, and you are responsible for every action you take that affects these things. Responsibility for your health begins with you, the patient. For a responsible adult in a free society, it can't be any other way.

A patient's duties start long before he or she goes to a doctor. Most of these duties are everyday activities. Though young children are exempt from this, as a child gets older, the obligations of health consciousness start, and from there they grow. Parents have always had a duty to teach their children basic healthcare skills—brushing teeth, bathing, cleaning cuts, avoiding colds, flu and other common illnesses, eating right, exercising, and so on. When we reach school age our teachers take on some of this responsibility, but they also act on the reasonable expectation that we already have a foundation of basic health training from home. Even when we are in kindergarten our teachers expect us to take some responsibility for our bodies. Among other things, we're supposed to dress warmly before going outdoors, excuse ourselves when we need to go to the bathroom, and wash our hands when we're done. We learn early, if something is wrong, we're supposed to tell an adult.

For adults health should always be a primary concern. We owe it to ourselves, and, if we expect to have access to our community's healthcare facilities, we owe it to those with whom we share those resources. It's like the uninsured driver from an earlier chapter: When he has an accident on a public road, wrecking property and harming people, he's using and abusing resources that affect us all. He's hurt the community. The injured people need treatment, and the damaged property must be repaired. We demand that the driver have insurance covering at least some of this. Though our bodies are our own, if we expect others to heal us, we must be responsible about ourselves. When someone intentionally harms his health, then expects the system to take care of the problem, that person becomes a drain on us all. It's one thing to suffer ills or injuries that couldn't be prevented. It is another to knowingly make them happen.

Most of us know the most common threats to health. Some of these are present in almost any environment. We can guard against them, but they are always there. These threats begin in the home. Germs fester on surfaces, tools lie around waiting to be misused and abused, while potential accidents lurk in every corner. We can eliminate some of these by normal home maintenance. Keeping a clean house cuts down on germs, and makes living a healthy life easier. Those living in a clean home are generally less likely to suffer injuries, and more likely to eat well. Personal hygiene can also guard against health threats.

The most obvious dangers that we can avoid lie in our behavior. Almost all of us are tempted by the traditional vices: cigarettes, drugs, and alcohol. If we drink to excess, smoke, or poke needles into our arms, most of us understand that the long-term devastation will far outweigh any short-term benefits. If we eat nothing but ice cream we know we'll put on the pounds. If we spend our days on the couch, we know we'll get rundown.

Whenever we choose between healthy and unhealthy behavior, we should realize that we'll be responsible for the results. Learning this lesson is a basic part of becoming an adult. A 12-year-old taking her first drag on a cigarette might not appreciate this responsibility. A 22-year-old accepting his first shot of heroin should, and, if at all possible, he should be made accountable for the consequences.

A patient with a genetic disease isn't responsible for her genes, but she does have the duty to take care of herself as well as she possibly can. If a cystic fibrosis patient hangs around in rooms full of smokers, she should expect her symptoms to worsen. Most of the adult illnesses a doctor sees have some component of patient responsibility. Every day hacking smokers, cardiac-challenged couch potatoes and chocolate-gobbling diabetics come into our offices. Some are more obvious than others, but these differences can usually be measured in degrees. Almost all of us have a bad habit or two. At some point we all become contributors to our own demise.

I realize that few people are going to stop eating chocolate, nor do you have to feel guilty every time you open a bottle of beer. Still, each of us has an individual responsibility to ourselves to keep our bodies reasonably healthy. Good health isn't exactly the same for everyone. An eternally slim person doesn't have to worry as much about weight issues as a patient who's obese. A patient with a bad kidney might have a strong heart, and vice versa, creating unique health regimens for both. But all of these people begin with the same basic principles. All must pay attention to their bodies, even if they concentrate on different things.

If we turn a blind eye to our health duties, we should, at the least, accept, and prepare for the consequences of willful self-abuse. We should be conscious of what we put into our bodies, and, if we want good health, we must avoid, or limit those substances that threaten our wellbeing. If you go to bed every night with a stomach full of Big Macs and chocolate sundaes, you shouldn't be surprised when you wake up in the middle of the night with a major stomach problem. If you smoke a pack a day, you know you're flirting with lung cancer, emphysema and cardiovascular issues.

Most of this responsibility is a simple matter of habit. A balanced diet, regular exercise, and everyday personal grooming and care, have always been the staples of a healthy lifestyle. If you have a fairly normal body, and do these things habitually, you can have that occasional ice cream cone, or after-dinner drink without worry or guilt. Either one might even be good for you, as long as you stay within reasonable limits. If you exercise regularly, you might not need to worry as much about fats and sugars. But if you drink yourself to sleep, or eat a big bag of chocolate chip cookies for dinner each night, your health will reflect these habits. That's when diabetes and cirrhosis of the liver turn into predictable outcomes. Though we all have the responsibility to provide adequate resources for treatment, it's your responsibility to use them. You've done it to yourself.

This isn't a fitness book, so I won't set out any detailed health regimens, but anyone interested in good health should have such a program. Some lucky folks have no difficulties with this. Their taste buds and energy levels are in perfect tune with health foods and workouts. For these folks proper diet and exercise hardly seem like discipline. Some people are born loving broccoli and yogurt. Some kids start working out before they can walk. But for most of us good health is more work than play, especially as we get older.

In the healthcare business this comes into sharp focus every January. For so many people that first morning of the New Year brings an array of grand resolutions. With the holidays over, a lot of us wake up ten pounds heavier, slightly hung over, with our stomachs churning like acid factories. We throw out the garbage from the last holiday feast, then swear off everything we've been ingesting—no more chocolate, beer, or chips. No more fatty meats or fried foods. From here on we resolve to do only good things: run, lift weights, do yoga. We promise ourselves that we'll stick to a Spartan diet: no fats, no sugars, no processed foods.

For healthcare providers this New Year's ritual has another meaning: you'll be in to see us soon. All of you who are making resolutions are our once and future patients. As you shake off those post-holiday blues, you might begin with an online search for health club memberships. Or maybe you got a workout machine for Christmas. This is when you're most likely to set it up. It's a moment when the whole population seems bent on getting into shape, and many don't have the slightest idea of how to do it safely.

Almost immediately some of these resolute patients wind up in our offices and emergency rooms. They've run without stretching, jumped without looking, and landed without benefit of padding. Sprains, muscle pulls, and broken appendages abound. Crash dieters faint dead away, or, if they manage to keep at it for a few weeks, they develop vitamin deficiencies.

Though nearly every published fitness program suggests that its users consult their doctors before they begin, few do. For women that's often the call they forgot to make. For men it's related to our mental block against asking directions. Ultimately no one of either sex thinks he or she needs a doctor just to do a few jumping jacks or cut a few calories. None of us are that old. Right?

Most patients aren't in the habit of asking their doctors about New Years resolutions, but doctors don't have any incentive to encourage such discussions either. If you start a new activity, but don't tell us about it, we don't advise you about it. Besides, in the modern medical business model, prevention provides few rewards. Not many preventative measures have billing codes, and even those that do, like smoking cessation, are seldom actually paid for by the insurance policies. There are no reimbursement formulas for the treatment of foolish resolutions. As a result we must deal with the consequences.

Real fitness is not a once-a-year activity. It's an everyday part of life. Every patient's health and fitness will be different, but certain basics apply to us all. We need to learn to listen to our bodies. That means paying attention to our inner perceptions. We must be attentive to what we feel, both good and bad. We must be aware of what we're eating and drinking, and how food and liquids affect us now and later. If I'm sensitive to caffeine, I must limit my intake of coffee. If I gain weight easily I should keep strict tabs on sugar and fat. If I'm prone to laziness I should rouse myself regularly to exercise.

Parents need to teach these habits to their children, and the best way to do it is by example. If dad and mom lead reasonably healthy lifestyles, the kids are more likely to follow.

In most debates about healthcare issues, health is discussed as if it were a commodity. If you listen to the arguments, they will all be couched in terms that make health sound like a product that's bottled in a factory, shipped to a warehouse, then finally winds up as an item sitting on the shelf of your local healthcare store. With its prohibitive price tag, this is one of those products they keep behind the counter under glass—the kind that requires either cash or a credit card (or, in the healthcare store, an insurance card) just for a chance to closely examine it. The problem is that this pricey and limited commodity is necessary for survival. Anyone who's stopped a serious infection with an everyday antibiotic knows just how essential modern healthcare is. It almost always costs more than we have in the bank, so our question is always the same: how can we make sure everyone can afford it?

This viewpoint isn't entirely false. Healthcare is a commodity: a product and service provided by skilled professionals who do it for a living. They must be paid. Their tools are commodities too. Whether the healthcare provider is wielding a Q-tip or an MRI machine, someone must pay for the tool, and whatever goes with it.

But healthcare isn't the same as health. Health is not a commodity; it is the mental and physical condition in which a person lives. When you come into my office I don't sell you health or give you health. What I provide is a way to measure, evaluate and repair your health. If you're sick or hurt, I offer expertise in helping you recover. If you're well, I advise you about methods for maintaining your health. Whenever possible I look at your past and present condition, and help you prevent future problems.

This last service usually goes under the name, "preventative care." Through much of the last two decades ideas about preventative care have played a central role in debates about overall healthcare costs. This makes sense. If we can spend a few dollars today to prevent a problem, that's obviously better than spending a few thousand dollars to deal with its consequences later.

But what is preventative care? Some of the best examples are what I've been writing about here: basics of personal hygiene. These are habits most of us learn as children. Washing one's hands before cooking or eating is one. Cleaning the bathroom and kitchen is another. Regular exercise is a preventative measure, as is eating a sensible diet. These actions help us avoid colds and flu, and keep our vital organs in shape. A sensible diet helps us replace and renew dying tissues, while giving us energy and stamina. If we add exercise to that, we build muscles, increase our overall strength, and reinforce our immune systems. That gives each of us a better chance of staving off everything from cardiac problems to cancer.

The first steps in prevention begin before birth. This is what's become known as prenatal care (a term that didn't come into common use until the 1950s). We all know that a pregnant woman who eats right, takes care of herself, and gets proper exercise is likely to have a healthier baby. Prevention continues after birth. That's when we start recommending certain vaccinations. Breast-feeding is another preventative measure. A mother's milk helps a baby build natural defenses against many illnesses. As a child grows up there are more vaccinations, and the child learns countless small preventative behaviors. He cleans up after himself, dresses warmly in winter, and wears sun block on bright summer days. The child will carry many of these habits into adulthood.

As we get older prevention becomes more complex. Though the same old habits still help, the emphasis shifts. Up until now we've been preventing hindrances to proper growth and maturity, but once we reach adulthood we focus more and more on preservation. We want to save what we have left, a task that gets more difficult with the years. As we pass from youth to middle age, preservation is the prod behind almost every New Year's resolution. With each year we want more years, and we want all of them to be healthy.

Prevention, as practiced by the patient at home, or in the course of normal living, is a valuable principle to follow. For as long as there have been people, some of us have been using common sense to keep ourselves healthy. Programs that teach and encourage these behaviors help keep patients out of ERs. But in healthcare coverage prevention can mean much more.

Many healthcare providers see prevention almost exclusively in terms of what can be done in a doctor's office or at a hospital. This approach is centered around testing. Some testing makes sense. Someone with a family history of colon cancer should start getting regular colonoscopies before others would. A patient with genetic markers for heart disease should start heart-friendly exercises and diet early.

When discussing excess testing, we need a few ground rules. Though some testing practices have gone out of control, testing for diseases and conditions is an essential part of medicine. Without it we would lose important data that helps us target drugs, therapies, and other treatments. When we apply the principles of logic and reason, today's screening and testing procedures work well. The problem comes when doctors, institutions and the demands of patients combine to broaden testing criteria to the point where nearly every patient gets screened for every problem—even those conditions that are nearly impossible. This gives us endless false positives, which often create a need for further tests. Somewhere in the process common sense dissolves into nonsense.

Take the electrocardiogram, or EKG. For decades this was our main test for heart problems. In most instances EKGs could detect whether a damaging heart attack had happened, though not always. Sometimes we saw the symptoms in the patient, but no signs on the EKG. Other times there were false positives. Over the years, as medicine got more sophisticated, we found other tests. When the EKG failed, we could measure the level of heart enzymes released into the blood. This created lot of false positives too, but it was also more sensitive and specific, allowing us to recognize many less obvious problems, such as small leakages of muscle enzyme. With today's procedures, if I have a major heart attack, that should show up on the EKG. If I have a minor enzyme leak that should be clear from a blood test. The events are both heart attacks, but they are two very different conditions. One is massive and life-threatening; the other is serious, but manageable. If I had a choice between the heart attack detected by the EKG and the leakage found by the leaking enzyme test, I'd take the leak any day.

Recently I saw an example of how misuse of these tests can lead to tragic consequences. A 35-year-old male patient experienced chest pain after exercising at the gym. His was admitted with a referral from his primary physician. He complained of pain that was confined to his chest wall. It hurt when he moved his arms or flexed his chest. As one would expect with a man who spends a lot of time in gyms, this man was in pretty good shape. At 35 any severe heart problems would have been unusual. Still, they were possible, and, or course, there was that chest pain.

What caused it? Pains can come from many sources. A cancer in the prostate might first announce itself with searing back pain. A brain tumor might cause pain in your arms or legs. Heart attacks can show up in the arms, legs, stomach—or in the chest. At the same time, we often experience similar pains from far less serious causes. We pay little attention to most of these, and if one fools us, prompting us to see a doctor, we feel incredible relief when we learn that it's nothing—*if* we learn that it's nothing. This man's chest pain might have come from a moment when he stretched too far, or bumped into something, or when something bumped into him. Or it could've been a serious cardiac issue. Without explicit markers there was no way to be sure.

By the time the patient finished getting his EKG he was already feeling better. That might've been the end of it, but then the results came in from his enzyme test. His enzyme levels were slightly elevated. This should not have seemed at all odd. His chest wall was still tender, and any injury can push up the numbers on enzymes. Unfortunately, the same is true of a heart attack. Still, with no known risk factors for premature cardiac disease, and (except for minor chest wall tenderness and slight enzyme-level elevation, each with far more probable causes) no apparent cardiac markers, he might've been discharged. The rest of the examination showed nothing to indicate a cardiac event. But his primary physician was not yet convinced. Though his patient's symptoms were quickly fading, the primary physician (who'd referred him to the ER in the first place) now admitted the man to the hospital for a more extensive evaluation. This was one of those times when further tests wouldn't help the patient, but no one knew that yet.

When a blocked artery causes chest pain, it's common to administer aspirin. In these cases we also often use nitrates, and we often give cardiac patients Heparin, an intravenous anticoagulant. Despite his low risk for heart attack, doctors started this patient on all three. As the patient waited for the next procedure, he complained of a sudden and severe headache. The primary physician thought the nitrates were responsible. He discontinued them. Over the next hour the patient's headache worsened. Suddenly he began having a seizure. A CAT scan showed a large intracerebral bleed. Blood was leaking into his brain. This was a rare, often devastating, but recognizable side effect of Heparin. The doctor stopped the Heparin immediately, but it was too late. The man's brain was damaged, and now his prognosis was a life with permanent limits. Further tests revealed no cardiac damage. The only real problem had come from the questionable test, and the unnecessary precautions it prompted.

The patient's doctor had been cautious. The ER doctors were cautious too. The examination was thorough—thorough enough to catch that mild elevation in enzyme levels. The treatment was cautious—so much so that this is a case where the doctors' behavior perfectly fits the phrase: "erring on the side of caution." In some cases to err on the side of caution means doing little or nothing, but in modern medicine it usually means more tests. Further caution means giving test results the worst possible interpretation, then acting on it. Modern medicine has little patience with a do-nothing approach.

What should have happened? It's always hard to second-guess, but it's clear that this man should not have received Heparin. The only reason he got it was because an internist feared the improbable possibilities implied by a test that probably shouldn't have been administered in the first place.

Instead the doctors should have looked at the whole patient: fit, 35, with no history of heart problems. They should have regarded him as a low-risk for cardiac issues in all their calculations. If clear-and-present evidence of cardiac issues arose, the patient was in a hospital, where they could address the problem quickly. But the basic assumption should have been that this otherwise healthy man had chest pains whose cause should be investigated. If the pains faded, the crisis was probably over. If they continued, then action would be taken. He should have been monitored, and when nothing else happened, he might've been given a stress test the next day, just to be certain. If this had happened, he would've been out the door and on his way. Instead excess testing and erroneous treatment left him with lifelong brain injury.

We have similar testing problems with diabetes. Where we once used a glucose tolerance test, we've replaced that with a measurement of the marker, Hemoglobin A1C. The new test allows internists to diagnose diabetes much earlier, but in many cases they are only finding the marker, and no other sign of an active disease.

Recently a woman arrived at the ER complaining about abdominal pain of several weeks duration. It was located in the upper epigastric region. It tended to affect her in the evening, after she'd eaten, though it also showed up after other meals. Her pain didn't seem acute. Her vital signs were normal, and she wasn't vomiting. This hardly seemed like an emergency.

The woman smoked, and admitted to being a social drinker. Occasionally she took ibuprofen. In her answers to standard questions the woman said she hadn't been traveling. She also reported no bleeding, fatigue, or recent illness. She admitted that she often got relief from taking antacids, but still she had a concern relating to her family's recent health history. Her aunt had just been diagnosed with pancreatic cancer after showing similar symptoms.

The patient wanted an in depth evaluation. At her request the doctors set out to do blood work and a CT scan of her abdomen and pelvic area. After being treated in the ED for presumed gastritis/esophagitis, she felt better. Her CT scan was coming up.

While getting the scan, something went wrong. When the "code blue" went out, several of us rushed to see what had gone wrong. "Code blue" meant that her life was in immediate danger. How had this happened? She'd had an anaphylactic reaction (a sudden, life-threatening allergic reaction) to the intravenous dye used to create contrast in CAT scans. Her airways had swelled, as had most of her body, and now she was suffering from asphyxiation. Unable to intubate her, we cut a surgical airway (tracheotomy), and managed to resuscitate her. But the damage was already done. The short period of anoxia (no oxygen) was enough to impair her brain. It was permanent. The patient would never return to a normal life.

This woman was suffering from acid indigestion— what we now call acid reflux disease. In the short run she needed nothing stronger than an antacid tablet or two, and in the long run other reasonably benign treatments were available. If we'd wanted to test her in a different way we might have run ultrasound, but even that would've probably been overkill.

Both of these patients were victims of overzealous testing policies. If a patient wants a test, we give it. Any patient we test might show disease markers. If the patient is truly ill, and we haven't agreed to test, or we ignore the markers, we could wind up being sued. So we test for all possibilities, no matter how far-fetched.

Much of modern science is based on a physics discovery called the Uncertainty Principle. According to this, you can't measure a thing or a function without altering it. In other words, the observer always changes the observed, no matter how small those changes might be. Like all other scientific investigators, medical researchers try to devise tests that have the slightest effects possible on the patient. Scanning procedures use as little radiation as possible. Chemicals are devised and selected on their ability to detect while remaining benign. But we can never escape two facts: we are observing, and in doing so, we are changing what's observed. Whenever you alter anything, there's always the chance that the process will go out of control.

The increase in testing creates loads of new information. This information goes into charts and calculations. These give us the data we were searching for, and so much more. We take all these facts and figures, and look for associations between causes, symptoms, markers, diseases, and other factors. Whenever we see something new, we name it. In this way we manage to invent whole new sets of maladies. We usually create a name to associate with our observations, then add a word like "syndrome" or "disorder." Most of these are nothing more than collections of symptoms and markers that might or might not have significant associations. We assume these associations have meaning. If the meaning isn't there in the science, we put it there in the name.

Two of the more famous disorders are both physical and mental: ADD (Attention Deficit Disorder) and ADHD (Attention Deficit Hyperactivity Disorder). Both started with children, which means doctors discussed the conditions with the children's parents. Both got names, descriptions, along with prescription drugs and treatments. As awareness spread, so did the disorders, and within a few years many adults were afflicted.

With ADD you have a hard time keeping your mind on things. With ADHD your attention deficit is complicated by the fact that you've got ants in your pants. That's what the "H" between the two "Ds" represents. It's not that these aren't real, recognizable problems, but they're nothing new. There have always been people who can't keep their minds on a subject, and others who can't calm down. It's worst in children. Most overt behavior problems are. Often the two conditions combine in one body. Then we have double trouble. We try discipline, soothing words, and other methods. We even give them sedatives, and prescribe exercise programs. Sometimes one of these methods works.

Today we give targeted drugs to patients with these disorders. In many cases the drugs were specifically designed for the malady. Sometimes they work. Do they work better than older methods? No one really knows. But these new diagnoses certainly sell a lot of drugs.

We might begin to solve this by altering the way we approach medical problems. Up until now we err on the side of excess. A cough might be cancer, while a chest pain might be a heart attack. When you enter a medical facility we'll test for both. A mild headache produces tests for a tumor, while a rash might indicate that it's time to test for Lyme disease. Should we do these tests? In many cases we should, but in many other cases it might not be wise. Tests make sense when there's a reasonable possibility of finding something wrong, or if we simply want a more complete picture of the patient's health. If odds against the problem's presence are millions-to-one, and other possibilities are far more likely, then the test should not be automatic. We should rule out the most likely causes before we test for the more exotic possibilities.

We should also be more suspicious of associations. Sometimes these can light the way. Other times they create false links between supposed causes and unrelated results. When we see an obvious association between a possible cause and a visible effect, we have reason to look more closely. If the association is precise and statistically accurate, we must pay attention. But maybe we shouldn't name this association until we can learn something of how the cause creates the effect. Then we'll know if it's a syndrome, a disorder, or a full-blown disease.

The patient is the ultimate monitor. Excess testing is driven by the fears of doctors and insurers. Doctors have learned to see every new patient as that potential case-in-a-million where they might get sued. Who will sue them? The patient. Patients tend to want everything their insurance will pay for. Many patients arrive in an ER or office, insisting on receiving specific tests. They've all seen cases where the patients suffered or died from things that were detected too late. They're determined not to let it happen to them.

But, just as a doctor should look at the whole patient, and not just one symptom, a patient must be aware of the whole healthcare picture. A patient should respect tests for what they are: procedures that change something to measure something else. They are not all benign or neutral. Tests require tools and materials. Some of these are potentially harmful. We all die sometime, and a few of us die (or are hurried toward death) by testing. As we discover effective new detection methods, we should carefully examine how they operate. Doctors must explain upsides and downsides so informed patients can make better, more educated decisions about treatment options.

When it's the patient's choice, she should decide whether to get tests on the basis of her own feelings, symptoms, and history. Tests should not be administered simply because they're covered by insurance, nor should the decision to test be driven solely by the law. A test should be done to detect and/or rule out conditions or threats. The patient is the buyer here, and if he or she wants every test in the book, let the buyer beware!

Chapter Twelve: You Are Here

You enter the insanity of our healthcare system before you are born. At this point you make your presence known as a condition within your mother's body. As soon as a mother suspects she's pregnant she usually goes to the doctor. Once she does that, she's in the system, and so are you.

Pregnancy and childbirth are among the clearest examples of how poorly our system works. The most cited statistic in any nation's health picture is its infant mortality rate. This measures the percentage of our infants who die before reaching their first birthday. Because the most obvious healthcare needs show up at birth and death, a nation's initial healthcare advances will usually be most visible at these junctures. As a result, changes in a nation's infant mortality rate (IMR) can tell us whether that country's health infrastructure has developed into the modern era. In 1860 America almost 1-in-4 babies died before the age of one. By 1950 it was 1-in-33. Today it's about 1-in-150.[*]

IMR is not a perfect statistic. Different countries calculate it different ways. The United States and some other nations count any newborn showing signs of life as a live birth. Some countries don't. Most developed nations have a much higher rate of premature births, and ours is one of the highest, which elevates our IMR. Without medical intervention most of our premature babies would die in the womb, or during birth. In many other nations these would not be recorded as live births, so they would not go into the statistics. In the U.S. the inevitable failures that accompany

---

[*] United Nations World Population Prospects: 2011 Revision

some of our efforts to save our most premature births sends our IMR higher. At the same time, in undeveloped countries many mothers in remote villages never report infants who die during, or soon after birth, which artificially lowers their IMRs.

In most nations these factors cancel out one another, leaving IMR numbers that give us a reasonably good picture of a society's overall health. The rate at a given moment only gives us a snapshot, but if we look at it over years and decades we can learn a lot. Is the country's IMR going up? Down? Is it stuck at an unacceptable level? How societies handle childbirth says a lot about how they deal with general health issues. As a nation the United States spends more money on healthcare than any other. Like any developed country, we put a lot of our health-related resources into pregnancy and childbirth. We're among the world's leaders in prenatal testing, medical technology and prenatal care. We have more neonatologists (specialists in problems of the newborn), and a better ratio of neonatal ICU beds to infants, yet overall our infants don't do as well as those of other countries.

Singapore, Iceland, Japan, Sweden and Finland all have IMRs that are less than half of ours. In every thousand births they save 4 or 5 babies that we don't. Slovenia, Portugal, and New Caledonia hold sizable leads over us. Greece and Spain might hover on the edge of economic catastrophe, but they save more babies than we do. Just ahead of us are Croatia and Cuba. We often talk about the plight of these poor, disadvantaged nations, but they could teach us something about keeping our infants alive. All of our money, beds and doctors are only enough to rank us at 34th in IMR among the world's nations.

How important is this? If a lot of babies are dying, many of the ones who live do so at a cost. They've been born sick, but they managed to survive. Their illnesses leave them with damaged organs, compromised immune systems, and shortened lives. The more babies die, the more mothers suffer from disease and malnutrition. If the mothers are sick and hungry, so are their families. That's why a high IMR almost always indicates an impoverished, primitive society.

We seldom think of the United States as a place of widespread poverty and hunger, and for most of us those conditions are remote. Nevertheless, they exist here. Our highest IMRs come from the poorest groups in our population. Our upper income IMR statistics compare favorably with those of nations with the lowest infant mortality rates. This is a reflection of the inequality of healthcare services available to our rich and poor.

IMR is a measure of more than simple survival. It shows us how families, villages, and whole societies are faring as they try to bring more children into the world. Our poor are like a nation within a nation. They lack money, education, and, of course, healthcare. They have the dead infants to prove it.

The United States once prided itself on its progress on this front. Up until the mid-20th century we were almost always among the top nations in saving our infants. We still pay far more than mere lip service to advances in infant health, but our efforts are difficult to measure, maybe because we measure so much. This is one more area where we screen, test, and retest. Our prenatal testing has grown to encompass all the known possibilities and probabilities of an infant's development. Our efforts range from non-invasive methods to prenatal intra-utero operations. These specialized, technical and prohibitively costly interventions barely dent the IMR, yet babies born by these methods make the news more often than infants dead from malnutrition or cold exposure. We celebrate our most complex successes while ignoring the failures brought on by our simple neglect.

Prenatal testing really got off the ground here in the U.S. in the 1950s and 1960s. That's when researchers discovered that women over 35 were more likely to give birth to children with Down syndrome. This genetic condition comes with easily identifiable physical markers. Those who suffer from it have physical disabilities and IQs that are about half of those of normal children. Once the link was established between a mother's age and a child's disability, obstetricians began urging pregnant women beyond their early 30s to undergo amniocentesis, a sampling of fetal cells from the womb. This invasive method of detection led to a high rate of complications. Doctors devised an alternative in the alpha fetal protein, or AFP test, which detects possible neurologic or spinal abnormalities. This doesn't have the physical complications, but it gives us a high percentage of false positives. Now we usually use ultrasound. Despite more effective testing, no reduction has occurred in the rate of Down syndrome. The tests tell parents that the syndrome is there, but knowledge is not a cure.

Down syndrome is only one of a number of abnormalities we can detect. Other conditions, such as Tay-Sachs syndrome and cystic fibrosis, have genetic markers we can see long before a baby is born. With this kind of testing, it would be foolish to think that parents would never consider the results when deciding whether to continue a pregnancy. This isn't something most prospective parents would advertise, and in most cases their doctors and other medical personnel won't ask. That makes it hard to reliably estimate how many parents choose abortion when they learn of these conditions. Their invisible decisions could be the beginning of a selection process that screens for defects, and encourages the aborting of the "unfit." Do doctors, as a profession, or all of us, as a society, want to offer this kind of "quality control" to prospective parents? On the other hand, can we avoid it?

In the 1950s there wasn't much public debate over what to do if a fetus showed abnormalities. Abortion was illegal in every state. Little could be done about any of the pertinent problems. Any therapies, drugs or procedures were aimed at marginally improving the condition of the fetus, or preparing parents to face the challenges of raising an afflicted child. That began to change in the early 1970s when abortion became legal nationwide. The availability of abortion coincided with the sonogram becoming a ubiquitous part of pregnancy. Now parents could see the fetus, with all its abnormalities.

If a woman finds that she's carrying a fetus with Down syndrome, or any other physical abnormalities, there's little to stop her from aborting it. The literature from the various health agencies never mentions abortion as a tool for selective breeding, but the potential is there. There's plenty of evidence that it happens, and as tests become more sophisticated, it will happen more.

Abortion is one of our nation's most contentious issues, with the debates filling thousands of books and articles. It's not my focus, so I will only address it in the narrow frame of this issue. When coupled with modern methods of detection, abortion is no longer a question of when life begins, or protection of potential life, or rights of women and fetuses. In these cases it becomes a question of how we see ourselves. Do we want parents to use these tools to design their children's characteristics? Are there ethical and moral justifications for weeding out human imperfections prior to birth? Prenatal testing brings these questions to the fore by making selective births possible.

In any selection process the rich would have the upper hand. They have the money to test, treat, and/or abort. They can make sure that every child from a rich family carries biological traits favorable to creating better minds and bodies. Poor women will have fewer tests, less knowledge, and more kids with problems. That should help guarantee that the rich stay rich and the poor stay poor.

But if there's one thing we know in medicine it's that there are no guarantees. Results are seldom predictable. Even if we ignore the ethical and moral quandaries of selective breeding, we don't have any idea how such a practice would affect individuals or the human population as a whole. Eliminating one problem sometimes just makes room for others.

For instance, sickle cell anemia is a terrible disease usually afflicting people of African descent. If we accepted the idea of selective breeding to eliminate the disease from the human gene pool we would abort all fetuses that carry it, right? But before we do that we might also want to consider that, in many cases the sickle cell gene also serves as a protective mutation. The sickling of blood cells moderates the symptoms of malaria, in many cases eliminating them entirely. Malaria has killed more victims than any disease in history, and makes many more lives miserable. Until AIDS overtook it in the 1980s, annual figures always put malaria at the top of Africa's killer diseases. Since then it's stayed a close second to AIDS, killing nearly a million people a year. Those who carry the sickle cell trait (one copy of the sickle cell gene, rather than two) avoid most of the anemia's symptoms, while the gene protects its carrier from most of the effects of malaria.

From these kinds of complications we can see the limits of testing. The information gleaned from any test is limited by what we're testing for. Like those doctors who look at a single symptom, rather than seeing the patient as a whole, we tend to see tests in isolation. We test for a particular cancer, and find it, but the test tells us nothing about what produced the cancer, or things in our physical makeup that might fight the cancer. We test for the disease, not the cure.

That's the state of the medical world the prospective mother enters. Once she's in the healthcare system, her providers are likely to recommend a variety of tests and procedures. Most women will want whatever their insurance covers. This usually includes sonograms, blood tests, and a great many check-ups.

As we've seen, every test is an opportunity for the system to create more problems than it solves, and in pregnancy, every problem is magnified. Is there a chance the child will be deformed? Is it possible he won't be able to play football? Might some imbalance keep her from graduating at the top of her class?

Logic tells us that it's best to solve problems early. Pregnancy and infancy seem like the sensible times to deal with any potential threat. That's when we can nip it in the bud, right? That's when the baby has no choice in the matter, so we're only dealing with our own ideas and desires. We assume we want what's best for the child. Otherwise what kind of parents would we be?

We begin with the notion of fixing these things so the infant can have a normal, ordinary life. As we begin tinkering, we learn about methods that do everything from increasing cognition, to staving off old age. As we agree to more tests and procedures, we approach a line beyond which our motivations subtly change. Once we exchange abnormally bad for normal, how long will it be before we're trading normal for abnormally good? Ultimately we will want perfection—or at least abnormally attractive.

From the first misinterpretations of Darwin, through Hitler's genocidal eugenics, and into the present, the prospect of selective breeding is terrifying and wrong. Its vision can be expressed in the ludicrous oxymoron: "perfected humanity." Its potential is for a human race that manipulates itself into extinction.

Chapter Thirteen: *"I Fought the Law and the Law Won…"*[*]

In an ideal world medicine and law would both be tools for health and healing. Medicine would strive to heal each patient's physical ailments, while the law would help settle differences, and ensure the public's safety and welfare. Wouldn't that be great?

So where is this ideal? You won't find it in law. The law manages to limp along well enough to give most of us a modicum of safety and welfare, but some would say it creates more differences than it settles. Americans like to sue each other. Increasingly we've created a body of laws and court precedents that encourage us to use courts to settle every dispute, no matter how trivial. The result is a legal system where a convicted Colorado kidnapper can file suit against his two victims for breaking an oral contract they'd made with him to help him elude police. In their answer the accused victims allege that their kidnapper used coercion. At last check that suit was still pending.

Just about all of us have some experience with lawsuits. If we haven't been in one, we know people who have. In America it's common for suits to split families, fracture businesses, and even reconfigure governing bodies. Many of us who don't think we've been involved with lawsuits, actually have been. Have you ever received a small check from a class-action settlement? Tens of millions of us have. That means you were a party to a lawsuit, and you

---

[*] *I Fought the Law,* by Sonny Curtis of The Crickets, Acuff Rose Music, 1958

won! No doubt you and your fellow plaintiffs made a law firm much richer, and you didn't even have to try.

Just about every American who works in a trade or profession knows something about lawsuits, as does any business owner. Though there are no accurate figures on how many suits are filed, recent surveys show that at some point in their careers over 90% of independent business owners, professionals, and trades people consult their lawyers due to threats of legal actions. Most come from customers, clients or competitors. Many of these disputes arise out of claims of malpractice: the client says the professional didn't do his or her job properly.

Technically "malpractice" applies to negligence, incompetence, or wrongdoing in any kind of work, but in recent decades its meaning has narrowed. Now most of us use it only when speaking of medicine.

The medical world I've been describing is far from ideal either. Though we can heal wounds, cure diseases, and alleviate the pain and misery of most of our patients, we work in a broken system that drives everyone—doctors, patients, and even insurers—crazy. It's a world where nothing adds up. Costs and prices have little to do with each other. Bills come in duplicate, triplicate, or higher multiples. When insurance policies don't overlap, causing multiple payments, they leave gaps wide enough to squeeze a bankruptcy through. It's a system where the rich pay less, the poor pay more, and half the time no one's sure who's paying whom except the one who's banking the money.

It might seem nonsensical, but there are some bedrock principles at work here. Unfortunately they're the wrong ones. The first is that all practitioners must achieve a failure rate of zero—there should never be a bad outcome. The second is that you can never have too many tests. Of course, these concepts are linked, and the connections between them show up in practice. Together they create an impossible ideal, and in the real world of sickness and medicine, that ideal remains impossible. We test and test to make sure we don't fail, then, if we do fail, we test some more to make sure it never ever happens again.

The result of these impossible principles is doctors' very justifiable fear of the law. Thousands of patients sue their doctors every year. Hundreds of thousands more threaten lawsuits. This wasn't true fifty years ago. There were malpractice suits then, but their number and nature wasn't enough to make a conscientious doctor fear for his license. That was before the med-mal litigation explosion. Doctors' groups, patients, and even some lawyers have criticized the whole framework of current malpractice law, citing an average 12% annual increase in malpractice costs since the 1970s.

"Failure" to run adequate tests, and the expectation of a zero failure rate in outcomes, are the main causes of this increase. The perception that there should be an absolute guarantee of successful outcomes is the crux of the problem. The most competent and conscientious doctor in the world can't guarantee that. Even if we were to erroneously assume that it was somehow possible, this amazing doctor would have to do whatever was necessary to keep all his patients alive and healthy forever. Then, on the day he died, his successful efforts would end. In death he would fail all his patients. If we apply the zero failure ideal, they would all have grounds to sue his estate for malpractice.

"Zero failure rate" and "ideal" are synonymous. "Zero failure rate" is self-explanatory: to achieve it is to achieve perfection—nothing ever goes wrong. The first dictionary definition of "ideal" says: "A concept of something as perfect."

Perfect. No room for failure, flaws, or even the slightest error. An ideal is a yardstick whose end we can never reach. We know perfection is unattainable. Instead we usually measure human achievements against that yardstick in an effort to come as close as we can. Ideals are simple, straightforward concepts that have no physical existence in our day-to-day lives. When dealing with actual human bodies, there is no such thing. Every patient is different. That's why we adjust dosages, and adapt procedures. In medicine the standards are often starting and finish lines, with treatment being the whole racecourse.

When a whole profession is forced to live up to an impossible standard, with steep financial penalties for every setback, that profession will soon be in serious jeopardy. That's what's happening in medicine today. This can be seen in obstetrics where a majority of practitioners have changed their working methods due to malpractice concerns. A recent survey showed that the change 8% of them made was to simply go out of business. [**] Many of these are fine doctors, but they've seen the writing on the wall. They know there must be more sensible ways to support themselves and their families.

A malpractice suit begins with an action or inaction. The action might be a procedure, or a treatment, or a course of therapy. It could be a prescription or simply some advice. As we noted earlier, it's often a test. Or it might be a combination of any or all of these things. The doctor does what she does, but it fails to bring the desired result. In a high-risk case the outcome might be death. Less lethal outcomes might be side effects as small as a few headaches, or as serious as lifelong paralysis.

[**] The Case for Medical Liability Reform, *American Medical Association*, 2011

Inaction would be a failure to do one, any, or all of the above actions. The doctor observes, and finds nothing. If she tests, she doesn't run every test. Could she run every possible test? Maybe, if there's time, coverage, and the patient consents. You can always do more testing. If the results of a test have the potential to predict a bad outcome, and the bad outcome happens, then a court will often find the doctor guilty of malpractice due to negligence. On the other hand, if she ran the test, and it failed to detect the problem, an effective medical malpractice lawyer can usually make a case that the doctor should've run the test again—or run another test that might show the same thing. The point is, if something bad happened, and if there were the slightest possibility of it being detected, the doctor should've detected it. If she didn't, she failed, and that's not only unacceptable; that's willful negligence. The doctor not only screwed up, she did it with intent. After all, it was her choice not to do more testing.

***

A recent article in *The New England Journal of Medicine* reported that 75% of doctors in low-risk specialties will face at least one documented malpractice claim in their careers. For doctors in high-risk areas it's virtually 100%.[***] My career has been dedicated to the high-risk field of Emergency Medicine, a specialty where lawsuits sometimes seem as frequent as patients. I've faced several suits.

At the start of a med-mal case the plaintiff's attorneys usually name every doctor and facility possible. If you were a part of the process, you're likely to get served, even if all you

---

[***] Jena AB, Seabury S, Lakdawalla D, Chandra A (August 2011). "Malpractice risk according to physician specialty". *New England Journal of Medicine,* **365** (7): 629–36.

did was put on a band-aid. As the case moves forward they drop any defendants who don't look beatable. These care providers have often spent time and money, and endured much of the nerve-wracking process, yet they get no compensation, or even an apology. (A plaintiff's attorney would tell us that either one might tend to compromise the plaintiff's case.) Early in my career I'd been involved in cases like that, but I'd always been one of many defendants.

The first mal-med case I ever faced in the role of primary physician (the doctor officially providing the care) came when I was working at a tiny community hospital on the east end of Long Island. It was a weekend when a young woman arrived with her life partner. This seemingly pleasant woman was in the early stages of pregnancy. After successfully conceiving with the help of in-vitro fertilization, she hoped this child would be the beginning of a family. She lived in Manhattan, and was already seeing a high-risk obstetrician there.

She had a history of ovarian cysts, and she felt this pain was similar to what she'd felt with those. The remainder of her exam was benign. Our facility didn't have access to ultrasound services on the weekend, and by the time we finished, the patient said she felt better. We sent her home with strict instructions to follow-up with her OB in Manhattan, or to return to us if her symptoms worsened that weekend.

Instead she went directly to a university hospital 50 miles away, where she entered their ER complaining about the same pain. A full evaluation was performed, including blood work, urine tests and ultrasound, all of which were negative. They discharged her with instructions similar to ours: she was to follow-up with her OB when she returned to the city on Monday, or return to their ER if the symptoms returned during the weekend.

She did see her OB that Monday, but it wasn't until five days later that the doctor made a diagnosis, finally getting it by use of ultrasound. It was an ectopic pregnancy (one outside the uterus) for which she was treated. Though the previous weekend all of her tests had come up negative, she sued all the doctors who'd seen her at both hospitals. According to her complaint, we should've made the diagnosis the weekend before, even though the tests hadn't detected the problem.

The case dragged on for two years. I had endless conversations with lawyers, other doctors, and those who were close to me. The first time this happens, you question yourself. Even when you've thoroughly reviewed your memory and the case records, and imagined every possibility, no matter how outlandish, you can't see anything you would've done differently.

I went through the facts over and over. I'd done what I could with the equipment at hand. She'd reported feeling better before she left. When she visited her own OB (who'd overseen her pregnancy, and knew its history from the beginning) there were points of comparison we didn't have. Medical conditions are dynamic, ever-changing things, and seeing the full arc of a case is essential to accuracy. Nonetheless, it was another week before the OB had made the actual diagnosis, and that had been done with ultrasound, which we didn't have.

After two years of intermittent worry and legal sparring, the patient became pregnant again, and delivered a child. This pulled the legs out from under her case, and she finally dropped it. In medical malpractice, the plaintiff must have four elements: damages, duty, breach, and proximate cause. This patient's pregnancy fatally weakened any argument she had about damages. When we'd seen her, the pregnancy was undetectable, which contradicted her arguments about duty and breach. That was enough, but we should also note that the fourth element, proximate cause, is often the most difficult, even in a strong case. Even if we hadn't had all of our evidence on the other points, her pregnancy proved her case groundless. When it finally seemed like it was all over the lawyers and I had a good laugh. After two years, I needed that.

Still, that wasn't quite the end of it. Although there was no negligence, the hospital faulted me for not recognizing this patient as a potential emergency. The charge was that I hadn't transferred her to the proper facility. The hospital board felt that I should undergo re-education on how to care for a pregnant patient. The course cost a few thousand dollars, which came out of my pocket. That was the first case aimed primarily against me. Like any ER physician, I knew it was highly unlikely to be the last. That might give you an idea of why some doctors think about chucking the whole thing.

In the several suits I've faced, only once have I had to testify as a defendant. I was being sued with a group of physicians, and it was in that role that I testified. I'd learned about the suit in the normal way. A stranger came in my home, smiled, shook my hand, and said: "Are you Dr. Kessler." When I said yes, he replied: "You've been served." I watched him hurry out the door, then I looked down at the papers in front of me. As I read them I felt dread tinged with weariness. It's a feeling almost every doctor knows.

In Emergency Medicine med-mal lawsuits usually have multiple targets, and this was no exception. The papers listed all the doctors, hospitals and corporations involved. In this case I'd been the attending physician. The attending physician's role varies, but this time it meant that I'd co-signed a note written by a physician assistant (PA) who'd seen the patient in the ER.

ERs are hectic places. The patients' emotional states range from upset to traumatized. The personnel are overworked and often begin to feel ragged in the first minutes of a shift. This PA was working in our ER's "fast track" area. Patients are sent into the fast track when, by triage, we determine their needs are less acute. The fast track system is designed for rapid treatment and release. Patients who go there often have the most basic ailments: strains, sprains, lacerations, coughs and colds.

This patient arrived in the fast track complaining of a headache. He appeared to be in no distress. His vital signs were normal and he didn't look sick. The PA took appropriate history, performed a physical exam and deemed the headache's cause to be a sinus infection, something we see a lot of every day. During his fast track visit the patient received blood tests, intravenous pain medication and intravenous antibiotics—what's sometimes called a "million-dollar treatment."**** It might've been more than I would've given him, but PAs often go overboard. The PA had prescribed antibiotics and analgesics, then sent the patient home with detailed instructions to follow up with his primary physician if the symptoms worsened.

The patient did go to his doctor, but a few days later he returned to the ER. His headache had worsened. There was no fast track this time. As a patient returning within 72 hours, he was a "bounce back" who was automatically bumped up to a higher level for evaluation. He went straight

---

**** A treatment that goes well beyond the basic requirements.

to the ER where he was examined by a physician rather than a PA. There he received another complete physical, along with blood tests, and a CAT scan of his head, which the radiologist read as normal. Again the patient was sent home. Again he was instructed to follow up with his primary physician, which he did two days later.

I was the physician who co-signed the first note and I remembered questioning the PA as to why he decided to give a guy with a sinus infection the million-dollar treatment instead of basic prescriptions and a discharge. The PA said the fast track wasn't busy at the time, so he'd maximized his precautions.

Two days after the patient's second ER visit, when he returned to his own doctor, his still-worsening headaches included dizziness and poor balance. In addition, the patient's wife had noticed that he was confused at times. The primary physician's documentation noted the fact that our radiologist had done a CAT scan that he read as normal. The primary physician continued the treatment devised by the PA.

Five days later the patient went back to his doctor with symptoms that had grown much worse. This time they were bad enough to prompt his doctor to call for an ambulance. As soon as the hospital admitted him, the physicians there did an MRI, and diagnosed a brain abscess. For the next few weeks he was on intravenous antibiotics. After that he moved to rehab, and ultimately he returned home.

Two years later I was served at my home. Like all doctors in this position, I examined the papers to see what it was all about, wondering what I'd done or hadn't done. I'd never met, or even seen this patient. I knew that neither the PA, nor the radiologist, nor I, had intended to do anything wrong, and obviously the PA had done everything that seemed necessary, and then some. At that point I did what all physicians do: I called my insurer.

When policyholders get sued the insurance company refers the case to an attorney. Months later you hear from him. He meets with you, reviews the case, asks about your role, and you both try to get an accurate picture of how the charges against you could add up to a malpractice case. You've already read the charges yourself. The wording in these would make anyone angry, but it's best to roll with the punch. The charging document states that you knowingly, intentionally and willfully harmed, injured, deformed, and scarred this person for life. According to the plaintiff, his daily suffering, and his loss of time, spousal comfort, and happiness is a direct result of your willful ignorance and deceit. This document had all of that, and more.

In most cases the insurance company will pay for the attorneys defending you. Most exceptions are cases your insurers feel are hopeless. In a case where your insurance company wants to settle and you do not, your choices are limited. At that point you must either retain your own counsel or get another insurance company. With multiple defendants, it's best to present a united front. One reason the plaintiff's lawyers have included so many names in their allegations is the hope that the defendants will have a falling out.

In this case the plaintiff was suing all parties, except the PA. Most likely this was his lawyer's call. A malpractice lawyer would know that while PAs are insured, their limits are usually quite low. The deepest pockets in most med-mal cases are the doctors and the hospital.

Prior to going to court, all defendants are deposed. The deposition process is one of the most unnerving situations I've ever endured. This one was done in the attorney's office, with a court reporter taking down every word. The reporter reminded me not to use head gestures or nods—to put whatever I wanted to express directly into the words. That's the only thing the judge would see.

The plaintiff's attorney began with my resume. He went way back. I don't recall exactly how far he probed, but I've heard of cases where accusers wanted everything back through high school. After awhile the guy agreed to admit I had an education, and that I was actually trained as a doctor. Once he'd satisfied himself about that, he began his questions. Had I read the accusations? Did I understand the charges? Had I reviewed medical literature pertinent to the case?

My attorney had prepped me for this. In my testimony I stuck to a "just the facts" approach, answering only what was asked. I avoided using vague terms like "standard of care," or naming any source as an authority. If you cite a source as authoritative, the lawyer may find something else from that source that softens your case, or even appears to contradict you. That's when you know you've shot yourself in the foot.

I'd familiarized myself with the case earlier, but the questions, and sparring between the lawyers, helped me focus on various details. The basic suit was simple. The plaintiff contended that the ER and his primary physician had missed the diagnosis of his brain abscess. The missed diagnosis led to a prolonged recovery, and permanent mental damages, as well as loss of income, family time and spousal comfort. The notion that we've robbed the patient of his sex life is always on the list. That's an indication of where our legal interests lie in this country.

As a defendant, I'd been allowed to review the primary physician's medical records. It appeared that no one diagnosed the patient's neurological symptoms until a week after we saw him in the ER. I saw that it really was an unfortunate case, and I reflected that the penchant many doctors have for prescribing antibiotics to treat sinus disease might be a fear of the infection extending into the brain. Though this complication is extremely rare, it does happen, and if it can happen, we must stop it before it starts... right? Whatever the case, the PA and I should've seen this brain abscess coming, no matter how unlikely. That was the plaintiff's logic, and it wasn't without precedent. That's the thinking that drives so many legal and medical actions today.

By this time I realized that, despite harsh language and sharp questions, the atmosphere in the room wasn't all that bad. There was no animus or contempt. My attorney knew the plaintiff's attorney, and they seemed to be on reasonably good terms. There wasn't much tension. I didn't like being there, but worse things had happened to me. I answered the questions, covered what I had to cover, and was glad when the ordeal was over. I sat through the rest, then got out of there. I tried not to think about the possibility of a courtroom trial, but in this case the plaintiff was determined, making it unavoidable.

In court my testimony came early. I said the same thing I'd said in the deposition, but this time the plaintiff's attorney was more confrontational. He had me on the stand in front of everyone here, including the plaintiff's family. Their eyes stayed on me throughout my testimony. Other experts testified, but I spoke to what had happened in our ER. Though the PA had treated the man, I'd signed the chart, and the assumption was that I agreed with all parts of the treatment. As any med-mal lawyer will tell you, this is a situation where a united front is essential. The plaintiff was suing (among others) the hospital and me. It was important that hospital personnel not contradict one another when giving evidence. Though the plaintiff's attorney tried to twist my words, I gave strong testimony, carefully explaining what had been done, and why. It must have worked. The plaintiff soon dropped us from the suit. His own doctor was another matter. The primary physician's deposition had been clumsy, and overall he hadn't been impressive. When the case dragged on, he agreed to pay an out-of-court settlement.

In all of these cases the monetary cost is measurable. What's much harder to assess is the psychological strain. Whenever some important juncture looms in a lawsuit, every stranger who walks into a doctor's office looks like a potential threat. The signs of strain—heaviness in the chest, rapid heartbeat, sweat, and all the rest—are undeniable.

So why did each of these patients sue? A brain abscess is certainly devastating and life-altering. The consequences can be tragic and permanent. An ectopic pregnancy could be an imminent threat to the mother's life. But both of these cases are examples of elusive diseases that often don't present themselves on the initial encounter. Despite the fact that both patients received competent and conscientious care, they had bad outcomes.

In our litigious society, when medicine isn't perfect, patients are encouraged to enter the medical lottery of malpractice suits. The woman caused a lot of grief, but got nowhere. In the end she had her baby. The unfortunate man didn't get all he sued for, but his doctor's fear guaranteed that the patient would get some kind of settlement. I was just happy that, in the end, we were dropped from his complaint.

Chapter Fourteen—Up Against the Board

Every state has licensing requirements for physicians. Each requires that state's doctors to comply with certain standards of education, experience, and ethical conduct. Most states have boards or commissions that enforce these standards. Board members and commissioners look at complaints, weigh evidence, and pass judgment.

In New York our primary enforcement mechanism is the Office of Professional Medical Conduct or OPMC. The OPMC investigates complaints, and reports its findings to its own State Board for Professional Medical Conduct. This is something like a court, but not exactly. If there are complaints about a physician's conduct, the OPMC looks into it, and the Board passes judgment. The Board can fine a physician, or restrict, suspend, or take away the physician's license. It is both judge and jury.

In 1999 I was a member of the Board, and a willing participant in the process of governing my profession. I believed the system worked reasonably well. It wasn't until years later, when I woke up one morning and found myself being judged, that I began to have doubts. The charges against me, and the results of my "hearing," left me with an entirely different viewpoint. That's when I realized how damaging and costly this Board could be for a doctor, even if he or she had done nothing wrong. While it was true that they could go after unqualified quacks who botched surgeries and pushed narcotics, they could also impose draconian fines while recklessly damaging good reputations. I learned this the hard way: by getting charged, tried and convicted.

Admittedly, my own case began with my own actions. What I did wasn't entirely smart, and, as I later learned, was not at all wise, but I didn't lie, nor did I harm anyone. My transgression began with need and carelessness. Looking to boost a sagging income, I answered an ad for a job reviewing documentation on cases at a rejuvenation clinic in the Bahamas.

The Bahamian doctors needed certain, specific, non-formulary compounds—medicines that are not mass-produced—that were available from a Fort Lauderdale compounding pharmacy (a pharmacy specializing in the manufacture of these medicines). In order to get these they needed a licensed U.S. physician to review the specific cases on their patients, then write prescriptions for the necessary compounds.

It was a situation that might have set off my radar, but everything I could see online, and in their documentation, seemed to be perfectly legitimate. Still I suspected my signature was the main thing they wanted, so I insisted on reviewing all documents on all cases thoroughly. Most looked completely legitimate, and once I'd reviewed them carefully, I signed. I agreed to their prescriptions for various treatments and drugs. Some of the drugs would have been over-the-counter here. Others were prescription drugs familiar to me. Then one day I saw documentation on a case where the prescription didn't fit the patient's problem. It was the first one I denied. I sent the denial to the clinic, then all communication stopped. They didn't pay me for the final set of cases, and they didn't send any others. As weeks and months passed, and I still heard nothing from them, I began to suspect that the clinic wasn't all it had seemed. I felt as if they'd abused my trust, but I was glad they were out of my life.

It was over two years after that refusal that my wife arrived home from work one day, and found a business card stuck into the crack between the front door and the doorframe. The name on it was "Richard Springer." The face of the card also gave Mr. Springer's phone number, email, and employer. He worked for the U.S. Justice Department, and more specifically the Drug Enforcement Administration, or DEA. On the back of the card Agent Springer had jotted: "Please call me."

I called the number, and a moment later I had him on the phone. "What can I do for you, Mr. Springer?" I asked.

"We'd like to talk to you," he said.

"We?" I asked. "So this is a DEA matter?"

"Yes, Doctor, it is. I'd rather not discuss it over the phone. Could you and I meet?"

Right at that moment I remembered the Bahamian clinic. Though it had been more than two years, that was the only thing I could think of that might attract the DEA's attention. At the same time, I worked in a hospital with many other healthcare personnel, many of whom handled prescription drugs, so it could have been anything. I was curious, but obviously I would have to wait to see him in person. "Tomorrow's a little tight," I said, "though if it can't wait, I could make time. My best day this week is Wednesday. Where's your office?"

"No need to come to the office, Doctor." He sounded almost alarmed at the idea. "Our schedule is a little tight too. Could we meet on Friday?"

"Sure. So you want to come to my office?"

"No," Springer said. "I know where your office is. There's a McDonald's not far from there." He named the location.

"I know it," I said.

He gave me a time, and asked if it would be all right. I said it would, and hung up.

It all seemed a little odd, but the card looked real, and it turned out Agent Springer was exactly who he said he was: a card-carrying DEA agent fighting the eternal war against drugs. The following Friday, as we drank coffee at the McDonalds, he indicated that I'd been right about his current target. He was scrutinizing the Bahamian clinic. He'd done some homework, and even had copies of the prescriptions I'd written. Our conversation went roughly like this:

"It looks as if they're doing some pretty irresponsible things down there," he said, then he went into what the DEA investigation was uncovering.

It sounded pretty bad, and I said so. "I'm not surprised," I told him. "They looked all right to me at first, but then when I contradicted them one time, that was it. They stopped sending me cases. I figured that one bad case might've been a test."

"Maybe," he said, nodding.

"If I'd approved that one they would've known they could send me more like it."

"That wouldn't be at all surprising," he said. "Doctor, it would be helpful if I had copies of your records."

"The documentation they sent me?"

He nodded again.

"Sure. I've got a file full. Do you want me to bring it to your office?"

He shook his head. "No. This is a good place. We can meet here again."

What was it with these guys and offices? I wondered. Do fast food chains put something in their coffee that's especially addictive for law enforcement types? Or is there something about law enforcement that makes people hungry for Big Macs and fries? I should've asked him, but I never did. Instead, I showed up the next time with copies of all my records. I had cases, scrip, payments... everything he'd asked for.

Agent Springer seemed happy with the haul. "Yes, this will help," he told me over more cups of McDonald's coffee. Maybe it was the coffee, or maybe it was Springer's affable attitude, but I felt as if I was becoming a part of law enforcement too. I was a witness for the prosecution, a citizen doing my duty, a doctor bringing my professional skills to the aid of justice. Agent Springer would add my evidence to his own research, and make these irresponsible people pay. Though I knew of no specific harm the clinic had done, Agent Springer's investigation had convinced me. I was already prone to dislike these people. They were frauds, and they'd tried to make me into their dupe. Together Springer and I would take them down. Without ever specifically saying so, he made me feel like a partner in this noble mission.

We finished our second meeting with a friendly handshake, and returned to our respective jobs. Then I didn't hear anything for months.

My evidence was one small set of actions in the much larger story of "medical tourism." It's been going on for decades, but during the global boom of the 1990s it mushroomed. In the Caribbean, and other offshore tourist areas, clinics spring up specializing in treatments for everything from shedding pounds to curing cancer. In some countries these "medical tourism" destinations have become an industry. That's why I had been leery of the clinic in the first place, and it was also my reason for insisting on full reviews. I'd made sure my approvals were entirely justified by the records I was given, but in the silence following my one denial of scrip, I'd realized that my worst guesses about the clinic might be true. This place was probably operating on the fringes of United States law.

That's why I was happy to cooperate. I couldn't see much of anything damning beyond the one questionable case, but I knew that, like medical researchers, law enforcement investigators needed to see a broad range of evidence before they could detect the full pattern. My cases might serve as points of comparison, or could contain information that would only be recognizable to someone with access to the bigger picture.

I was plenty serious about going after the clinic. I felt that they'd duped me, then tested me to see whether I would stretch my principles. When I hadn't they dumped me fast. I'd felt used and abused, so I welcomed this chance to nail them.

***

The year before I reviewed the cases for the Bahamian clinic, my first boss had approached me about doing some work for New York's Office of Professional Medical Conduct. They needed physicians to sit on board hearings and advise lay members and the judge advocate about the medical aspects of the cases. My boss said the doctors they had tended to be older physicians and retirees. The Board was pushing to recruit younger doctors, who might bring a more up-to-date perspective to the work. It would only be an occasional case, the Director assured me, and it would be a good experience for a young doctor.

I agreed, and when I applied they took me. Over the following months and years I only worked on one OPMC matter. It was the case of a surgeon who'd been charged with inadequate care. The case went on for some time, and I wasn't there for the finish, but I did get a look at how the Board works. Even before I left I began to see the role the Board was carving out for itself. It was becoming a fallback mechanism for any case where malpractice could not be proved to a court's satisfaction, or any matter not quite within the range of normal med-mal procedures. In the end I wasn't happy about the way I had to leave the Board; nevertheless, when it came time to do it, I was glad to go.

In the months after I'd met Springer, I went on with my work, and he went on with his. Did he do anything to nail the clinic? I never saw any evidence of it. What I finally did see was his efforts to nail me. Somewhere along the line, probably long before Springer wedged his business card in my door, he and his DEA colleagues had chosen their target. As they were making that choice, the clinic probably didn't tempt them much. It wasn't within their jurisdiction, and with all the other international difficulties inherent in such an effort, they no doubt dismissed that idea early. But the clinic, and its relationship with the compounding pharmacy, would've turned up the names of American doctors, mine included. There I was, a licensed physician in the state of New York. I was available, cooperative, and accessible for trial on whatever charges they could think up.

At first the DEA didn't charge me with anything. Instead they gave the documentation from Agent Springer's investigation to the OPMC. No one told me about it. The evidence I'd given Springer to use in his investigation of the clinic was now being used against me. Those records were the basis of the complaint to the Board. It wasn't from a patient, or clinic, or a close colleague. It was from a federal agency whose agent had led me to believe I was helping him catch bad guys.

Once they informed me of the charges, I had to resign from the Board. One who's being judged can't be a judge. They found what they were looking for in the paperwork I'd provided to Springer. There they uncovered the fact that I'd prescribed human growth hormone and certain anabolic steroids. Studying the patient records, I'd felt these drugs were appropriate in every case I'd approved.

Though I hadn't been aware of it, these were controlled substances under the purview of the DEA. "Controlled" is not the same as "prescribed." When a substance is "controlled" the FDA puts some extra regulations on it. This happens with any drug that could easily be abused, or could cause serious harm or death. A variety of medicines and drugs fall under one of the five categories of controlled substances. Each category has an increased potential for abuse. The actual drugs range from mild painkillers, like Tylenol-with-codeine, to narcotics such as heroin and cocaine. This charge also meant I'd written the prescriptions on the wrong pad. According to New York law the drugs I'd prescribed required a triplicate prescription form, and monthly submissions of these records. I had used the regular forms that go with non-controlled substances.

I'd prescribed hormones and testosterone for individual patients, but the patients paid their fees to the clinic. The clinic then paid me on a per-case basis. I'd seen my role simply as that of a medical consultant for the clinic. Though I was reviewing individual cases, it was the clinic that sent me my paychecks, so that's what I thought of as the fee. But the DEA, and then New York's OPMC, decided to view this in a different light. They regarded the patient's payment to the clinic as the only fee. Using this premise, their logic was that if the clinic paid me a part of that fee, it was fee-splitting. Fee splitting is illegal in the medical profession, so that served as their basis for action.

When I saw the official complaint I was astonished. It listed 98 counts concerning 16 patients. Much of the wording was ominous. If one were to believe their version I'd been cavalierly passing out needles, syringes, and dangerous substances to anyone who wanted them. According to the allegations, I'd prescribed all these things without looking at the patients' histories or current records. My accusers alleged that I'd been subjecting these patients to "increased risk of morbidity and mortality," but that could describe a risk no greater than that of a 16-year-old girl getting her nose redone. They didn't cite any damage, or mention any ill effects to the patients. They just rammed it home that I had done wrong. Though I'd reviewed these cases carefully and individually, the charging document created an impression that I'd rubber-stamped every prescription. The real rubber-stamp was in their allegations. The charges listed regarding each patient were virtually identical. They substituted a letter for each patient's name, running from A to P. The only difference the charging document showed between most of these cases was this letter designation. That's really all they knew. There was no indication that they'd questioned any patients, and none of the patients had made any complaints.

If the patients were satisfied, and there was no indication of bad outcomes, what was the problem? Why were these people even interested in coming after me? A psychologist might have seen it as a kind of institutional "displacement." A slick politician would have known it for what it was: that age-old diversionary tactic we've come to know as "the witch hunt."

Though my case had occurred around 1999 and 2000, it didn't come to the Board's attention until 2004. By that year the steroid issue in sports was just heating up to a boil. Rumors and allegations surrounded some of sport's top performers, including Lance Armstrong, Sammy Sosa, and dozens of others. Star players sat before Congressional committees, their heroic auras wilting as they confessed their sins. Many of those who didn't confess took refuge in the Fifth Amendment. While pro sports tried to clean up its image, medical regulators nationwide worried that our profession would take a hit too. Their response was to see any case involving steroids as an opportunity to show that the medical establishment could police itself. They needed a live doctor who'd prescribed "performance-enhancing" drugs, and the presence of an offshore clinic didn't hurt either. It didn't matter who was getting the drugs, or why they were being prescribed. All that really mattered was the now-familiar phrases and acronyms like "anabolic steroids" and "HGH." As long as those were in the picture, my accusers were golden.

New York's OPMC website says the office "investigates complaints about physicians, physician assistants and specialist assistants and monitors practitioners who are subject to Orders of the State Board for Professional Medical Conduct." Though a physician's license is issued by the Board of Education, the OPMC, which is part of the Health Department, can revoke that license. These determined accusers could take my job and profession from me in a single action.

My lawyer reminded me of this as we drove up to Albany for the hearing. My med-malpractice policy had taken care of his fee so far, and ended up covering $25,000 of the $26,000 legal cost. Funny how those things match up. But as we drove north I wasn't thinking about the fee. All I could think about was how angry I was at these people.

"Be humble," my lawyer said. "You're not going to get anywhere with them, so your best bet is to just admit an error, and ask for mercy."

"But I didn't do anything wrong."

"You didn't actually see the patients in your office," he said, echoing one of the charges.

"That's true," I said, "and with telemedicine that's often the case. Besides, doctors are constantly working on cases where they don't see the patients. Another doctor, or maybe a PA, sees the patient, works up the chart, prescribes treatments or drugs, and later the physician in charge reviews it and signs off on it. This happens every day in ERs."

"I'm just saying you need to be calm, collected and contrite," he said, "and humble."

"But the whole thing is so flimsy," I said.

"It doesn't matter," said my lawyer. "This isn't a court. You don't have the same rights here. You don't have any right to discovery, or to a jury of your peers. All you get is an opportunity to speak. You can rant about your innocence, and the injustice of it all, but when you do, it'll be like punching these people in the nose. They'll get back at you. If you're not careful they'll take your license. Maybe you could appeal, but that would bring you up before the administrative review board—the same kind of panel you're facing today. And if you think this is costly..."

"Yeah," I said. "I see."

He was right, and I knew it. I was only talking about things like truth and justice because I was mad. I was mad because I knew the last things I could expect to find at this hearing were truth and justice. The only reason to go through it was to hold onto my license, and salvage my reputation. It was a balancing act: I had to be contrite enough to be a credible scapegoat, but I couldn't let my contrition go too far. That might encourage them to go overboard. When witch hunters get carried away, anything might happen.

My tribunal was made up of a judge advocate, two lay people, and two doctors. The doctors had the same job I would've had if I'd remained with the Board: they would advise the others and answer any medical questions. The lay people would decide whether I was guilty or not. The judge advocate would make a final decision on what the penalty would be.

When I saw the layout I was glad I'd never had to sit in judgment there. The Board sat at the end of a long table. I sat at the other end, my lawyer at my side. In between sat a physician reviewer. He would present the case against me. It was an inquisition-style setup, and I wouldn't have felt a whole lot more comfortable sitting with the inquisitors than I did as one of their prey. My judges didn't voice any such qualms. They had me where they wanted me.

In a courtroom trial we have the right to confront our accusers, but who were my accusers here? The patients at the Bahamian clinic hadn't accused me of anything. The people running the clinic never complained to anybody. Their only problem had been my refusal to rubber-stamp their decisions. My only real accusers were right there at that table in Albany: the Board. The physician reviewer would present the case against me, but he was really no more than the Board's representative. They board members were the power behind the charges. The Board had called me up on these charges, and now they would decide whether they'd been right. The physician reviewer's task was to tell them (and me) all the reasons they'd been right. Once they confirmed that they'd already made the correct decision, they would then make the real decision: what penalty I should pay.

The physician reviewer played his role to the hilt. Accusing me of misconduct and incompetence, he described my work as nothing less than handing out steroids and HGH to anyone who asked for them. He harped on the fact that I'd never physically seen these patients, making it sound as if there was no basis, documented or otherwise, to judge their conditions.

I might've asked him whether the Board took action against every physician who signed off on a prescription without actually seeing the patient in the flesh. I didn't. Instead I remained humble, while putting a few questions into the record. The physician reviewer was trying to cast doubt on the connection between the prescribed drugs and the documented symptoms. He made it sound as if I hadn't even glanced at the documentation. I might've noted that he was doing the same thing he was accusing me of: relying on the clinic's written records, rather than in-the-flesh observation. I didn't. Instead I simply declared that I'd felt I was taking appropriate actions. I noted that medical history is that of an evolving understanding of what we do. Treatments once thought to be effective, are now considered harmful. Others that we've never considered before, come into existence because someone notices a side-benefit, then incorporates it into practice. Many such treatments are now completely accepted by virtually all medical authorities.

My arguments didn't sway them. In the end they reached their pre-ordained verdict: guilty. I was a doctor writing steroid prescriptions at a moment when the public saw anything involving steroids as criminal. I was caught in a perfect storm. Investigators were probing sports ranging from track to baseball to bicycling. Fans were losing their heroes. Every night on the news we were seeing our sports stars brought low as they 'fessed up either to steroid use, or to the lies they'd told about it. As one athlete after another went down, investigators and prosecutors basked in the glory that comes with bringing the mighty low. Magistrates, judges and administrators gave in to the temptation to share in that glory. It was a decision that gave them the carrot while helping them avoid the stick. That year if someone in a position of authority didn't loudly oppose all "performance enhancing" substances, he or she was seen as being a part of the problem. The slightest whiff of sympathy for the accused could damage, or even end a career. The Board members were terrified of appearing soft on steroid use. I was a handy whipping boy. The verdict was inevitable.

Whipping boy or not, I was still a doctor. I'd earned my license through decades of honest effort. I'd done well in school, and practiced my profession honorably and competently. I couldn't let them take all that away. Staying within the bounds of humility, I said what little I could in my own defense. Though they found me guilty of threatening patients' lives and wellbeing, and of intentionally ignoring medical ethics and standards, they didn't take away my license. What they did do was to reprimand me, fine me, and restrict me from prescribing anabolic steroids and human growth hormone. They required me to swear I wouldn't do it again. They then made the entire record of their charges public, along with their harshly worded final judgment. That way any layman who read it would wonder how the Board could allow a monster like me to walk the streets.

When I left there I felt that the experience had a single, thin silver lining: the case had forced me to resign from the board that had just judged me. That alone left me feeling cleansed. But I still hadn't fully served the Board's purpose. That only came home to me the day after the Board's decision. Though I knew the decision was a part of the public record, I didn't think of it as being news. After all, there'd been no media interest up to then. The morning after the verdict was officially issued, that changed.

I was leaving for work, when I looked outside and saw the cars. I didn't know exactly who was in them, but they had the look of media. It turned out they were from the *New York Post* and the *Daily News*, two of the most influential papers in the biggest media market in the country. Someone had alerted them, and they were ready. Luckily my mailman drove up, and parked his truck in a spot that blocked their sightlines. I was able to get out to my car, and drive off before the reporters could intercept me.

I paid with incalculable damage to my reputation, and with a big chunk of my bank account. My lawyer cost me about $1,000 over what my insurance company covered, but that was small change. The DEA's parent entity, the Department of Justice, filed a civil suit against me. My acceptance of the OPMC ruling killed any chance for an effective defense against the feds' charges, and I wound up with a fine for $17,500. I also had to submit my scrip books on controlled substances for scrutiny every month for three years. That's what my eager cooperation had gotten me.

I'll readily concede that my views about the OPMC are biased by my own experience, but I'll also argue that what I saw there fits right into today's dysfunctional medical environment. The Board examined my case, allowing only limited evidence, then considered that evidence in a vacuum free of many of the constraints of normal legal proceedings. Once it reached its guilty verdict, it imposed sanctions and a fine, while making its selection of evidence public.

Like the medical professionals who run a million-dollar battery of tests on a dying woman with a spot of blood in her diaper, the Board looks only at one part of the evidence, and not at the whole picture. Just as the dying woman's doctors ignore her overall condition, the Board pays no attention to context of its charges. If the doctor was duped, it doesn't matter. If a doctor acted conscientiously and competently, that's immaterial. If they can find a charge that will stick, that's all that matters. With an excuse like that they can hold you up as an example, proving to themselves and the public that the medical profession isn't afraid to put the screws to any doctor, no matter what he or she has done. That's an awfully good picture of something we've all seen before: the witch hunt.

Chapter Fifteen: Birth and Rebirth

It was the kind of perfect Long Island day you sometimes get in the spring. The gray winter skies had finally given way to a warm blue preview of summer. A slight breeze carried scents of a thousand flowers. It was a perfect day for a birth.

Apparently nature noticed that, and not too far from our hospital Amelia Young (names here are changed) woke up to labor pains. The pains had been there the night before, but they hadn't been sharp enough for her to know whether they were real, or just more false alarms. She'd been feeling them for over a week. Before they'd gone to bed she hadn't mentioned the pains to her husband, Joe. She'd wanted him to get a good night's sleep.

It was when she woke up to that suddenly blossoming morning that she knew: this was no false alarm. She poked her husband, and said: "Wake up, Joe."

He stirred, opened an eye, and said: "'Nother fifteen minutes?"

"Not today. It's happening. We have to go to the hospital, and fast."

That's the picture I have of how their morning must've started. I don't know if it's entirely accurate, but it goes with what I saw fifteen minutes later. That's when I got to know these two pretty well in a very short time.

Between the moment they woke up, and the time they arrived at our ER, Joe would've discovered that he didn't have time to shower, or to have breakfast, or even to pull in somewhere for a cup of coffee. He would've learned these things because of what his wife was quickly discovering: this baby was in a bigger hurry than she'd guessed.

As Joe brushed his teeth Amelia informed him that he wouldn't have time for a shower. She was just hanging up the phone after talking to her obstetrician. When she'd told her doctor what she felt, he'd told her to get to the hospital immediately. "Go straight to the Emergency Dock," he'd said. "I'll get there as fast as I can."

The baby's insistence on coming out must've been the main topic of Amelia and Joe's conversation on what was surely a hair-raising drive to our ER dock. As they sped down the highway she would've begun insisting. The baby would've been insistent too, but Amelia had the voice.

We'd gotten word from her OB, but by the time his call came, Joe and Amelia were almost there. A tech out on the ambulance dock saw them speeding in from the street. He came inside, grabbed me, and said: "You better come." As we ran to the dock, he panted: "They just pulled in, and from the look of her, she might have it right there in the car."

As we reached the car I got my first sight of the situation. There sat a Lexus sport coupe, doors open on both sides, and a frantic driver looking this way and that, as he tried to figure out what to do about his wife. She lay all the way back, with her legs up, spread-eagled, and her feet planted on the dash. Her body knew what to do.

Like any ER physician, I've delivered my share of babies. I've seen slow births, fast births, ones with complications, and ones that went smoothly, but I'd never seen one come out quite like this. At the exact moment that I leaned into the car, the woman pushed, and the newborn did the rest. A baby girl popped out so fast, she literally landed in my outstretched hands. I should've been wearing a catcher's mitt.

A moment later I cut the cord. The tech had run back inside for towels, and now he started handing them to me. I tied the cord, cleaned up as well as possible, wrapped the baby in towels, then got mother and child into the hospital where the OB could take over.

It had been beautiful, and it had been quick. The place of birth was exceptional, as was the speed, but otherwise everything was normal. Helping a baby into the world is often much smoother than we expect it to be. In most cases the babies are ready. The mother's body knows what to do. The rest is just a matter of helping things go the way they should. A large head sometimes needs help getting out, or a caught shoulder might require some adjusting, and someone should be there to catch the baby, but otherwise the mother and child do most of the work for you. This changes only when there are complications. Those are the only times when modern medicine becomes indispensible. Women have been having babies for a lot longer than doctors have been delivering them. That's how we got here. My biggest role is to make sure nothing goes wrong.

Whether a birth is easy or difficult, when it ends with a normal little boy or girl, I see the result, and know why I became a doctor. Life is the most precious thing we have. I can't imagine a better job than helping it be the best that it can be.

That's the ideal medicine: promoting life. We can't always do it perfectly, but we do it every day. It's our job. Traditionally that's meant two things: making life better, and making life longer. In the past these goals seemed complementary. If we could cure an ailment, the patient usually recovered, got up from bed, and went on with a normal, or close-to-normal life. If an illness was terminal, we did our best, made the patient comfortable, and then the patient died. The first goal hasn't changed, and won't change. We strive to make life better. But in the last half-century the goal of extending life for as long as possible has been called into question. Too often this goal produces nightmares.

We measure health in many ways, but two criteria are always there: birth and death. These are moments where healthcare providers have always had a place. Long before there were gynecologists or obstetricians, midwives passed down the knowledge of how to help babies into the world. At the same time witch doctors, shamans and medicine men provided treatments and concoctions to heal afflictions and ease pain throughout a patient's life. When death came, they did all they could to make the final exit as painless as possible, just as Marcus Welby would. These early healthcare workers didn't have miracle drugs, or machines, or modern screening techniques, but they knew their jobs. They were there to help recovering patients return to a worthwhile life in this world, while soothing and comforting those who were headed for the next life.

No one likes death. Survival is hardwired into us. But death is a part of every life. A society that can't accept death blinds itself to one of the defining realities of life. There comes a point when it's time to let go. Sometimes it's simple. A patient felled by a massive heart attack dies without ever knowing what hit him. A bullet rips into a victim's heart, and she dies before she hits the ground. But most deaths are more complicated. Our powers of life extension have guaranteed that. A terminal patient in a modern hospital can often seem immortal. We put in the tubes, hook up the monitors, flick the switch on the ventilator, and until a responsible party tells us to pull the plug, we can often keep a body going indefinitely. If complications arise, we can usually deal with them. With the patient right there we can do whatever it takes to keep the blood pumping. The financial cost is sky high, and the emotional toll is incalculable, but letting a patient die violates some of our most hallowed traditions. We still feel we must say: "Where there's life there's hope." We are only beginning to ask the obvious question: "Hope for what?"

If we begin at death and work backward, we are starting from the most expensive, emotional, and irrational point in our healthcare system. In the U.S. 1% of the population consumes 21% of our healthcare dollar. Nearly a third of our Medicare dollars are spent on the last year of life. For a lot of us the last few days of healthcare will cost more than all the years leading up to that. Many terminal patients are comatose and will never wake again. We give lip service to hope, but in far too many cases we're keeping these patients alive simply because we can't face the responsibility of allowing them to die. It's as if the act of giving patients life, no matter how empty—automatically shuts off the possibility of allowing them to die—ever.

While these warm bodies consume the costly and finite resources of an ICU, young, conscious, uninsured patients go untreated. This is just one of the many irrationalities that makes ours the most expensive health system in the world—and possibly the most inefficient. We spend more money, give more treatments, produce more drugs, and concoct more therapies, yet we're not as healthy as many of our more parsimonious neighbors. Why? Because we have a system that's been out of control for decades. We're paralyzed by this self-perpetuating nightmare.

Any real solution will start with us. By that, I mean all of us: physicians, patients, insurers, hospitals, researchers, and every citizen. We'll end up doing it together, but the only way for that to start is for each of us to act individually. If enough of us make better decisions, our actions will bring us together. If the healthcare establishment finds itself serving a populace that demands rationality, efficiency, and humane treatment, the system will be forced to respond. Most healthcare professionals would welcome this kind of development.

We still think of medicine the same way Dr. Welby did. Doctors cure illnesses, heal wounds, save lives, and fight death to the finish. Doctors must be ever vigilant. When death threatens, the doctor acts. The same rules apply to all of us. We might not go to medical school, but if we can save a life, we know we should. In a life-threatening situation all other concerns are secondary. That was fine a century ago, or even in the 1950s, but for doctors, and other healthcare workers, it was changing even before Dr. Welby retired. The 1970s saw the first major end-of-life cases enter our courts. Forty years later we're still trying to sort this out. When does life end? No one knows. When should life end? We would like to think: Never.

An ideal of immortality requires that everything always work correctly. Otherwise there will be mistakes, and eventually one of these will be fatal. So our error rate must always be zero. The application of the zero failure rate standard to life-and-death situations is absurd. Death happens to everyone, and that will always be true. Yet, despite its impossibility, the notion of a zero failure rate doesn't stop there. Life-and-death situations usually develop out of less devastating health problems. But if those smaller issues can lead to life-and-death crises, then, in the interest of the zero error rate, they must always be avoided—*always*. And whatever minor irritants might lead to the smaller health problems must also be avoided...*always*. It's the kind of thinking that invites us to believe in the impossible, and when we can't get the impossible for free, we assume we can buy it with cash or insurance benefits. It makes no sense, but to think differently we would have to give up our ideal of immortality.

So it's here that I must come back to what I said at the beginning: We all die. Though many of us believe that our souls are immortal, our bodies are not. Our bodies die. We might have money or insurance, but we're still going to die. We could be in perfect health today, but eventually we will die. We can eat the right foods, follow rigorous exercise programs, find the secrets to health and wealth, or even discover the elusive fountain of youth—but we're all going to die. Acceptance of that basic fact is the beginning of rational thinking about healthcare.

That doesn't mean we should ignore healthcare, and give up at the first sniffle. It means we should tailor our healthcare to help us live the best lives we can. Avoidance of death should always be accompanied by a revival of conscious life—or, at the very least, a discernable chance for that. Our healthcare system should cure diseases, heal wounds, and help us live with disabilities. When those disabilities extend to a complete shutdown of thought and human consciousness, and there's no rational expectation of recovery, then we must learn to let go. This idea, and the catharsis of emotion it inspires, should become the basis of our end-of-life decisions.

Similar principles of humane rationality should apply to other health concerns. We have every right to expect our caregivers to be competent and informed. We should require them to always do their best. We shouldn't expect them to be perfect.

The closer death comes, the higher the price tag. We all want immortality, and as the end approaches we give no thought to cost or quality. Just keep the heart beating, we say. Who pays? Insurers, both public and private. Ultimately they get the money from us: taxpayers and policyholders. We pay every month, or quarter, or we have it deducted from our paychecks. It's the bulk of our second biggest household expense, an expense that will be first by 2016.[*]

Without insurance the situation changes. In most states if a homeless patient, with no family or contact people, lies stabilized, but with virtually no cognitive function, the hospital has clear procedures for pulling the plug. These procedures aren't sudden or automatic. Doctors examine the patient, and all pertinent information. Often an emergency ethics committee is convened. However, once these steps are taken, if the patient's case is hopeless, humane principles prevail, and the machines are turned off.

Insurance is our great enabler in our pursuit of irrational goals. We've come to see health insurance as a bottomless well providing money for anything health-related. Whether we want a heart transplant, chemotherapy, or round-the-clock intensive care, we expect insurance to pay. If we demand annual checkups and regular screening for scores of diseases, we expect insurance to pay. If a new ED pill is available, we want our policy to cover it. If women want bigger breasts, we insist that insurance pay for that too. We all want to pay an easily affordable premium that covers everything... *everything*. We don't want deductibles, we don't want co-pays, and we simply won't stand for any mistakes. We just want the medical miracles without any fuss.

---

[*] The Family Healthcare Budget Squeeze, by Christopher J. Conover, *The American, the Online Magazine of the American Enterprise Institute*, November 14, 2011.
http://www.american.com/archive/2011/november/the-family-healthcare-budget-squeeze. Accessed 6/11/2012.

We're quite serious about this. Anyone who doubts that need only look at our courts and TV ads. Those tell the real story of all our wants and desires. TV ads paint a picture of eternal youth and vitality on one side, and the vengeance of the law on the other. Drugs, therapies, and surgery offer us infinite pleasure right here on Earth, but if we don't get the treatment we want, we sue. If a doctor misses anything, even something that's not yet detectible, we sue. If a doctor doesn't specifically inform us of every potential repercussion, no matter how improbable, we sue. If the doctor we go to lacks every modern screening device, or the newest drugs or therapeutic equipment, we sue. If an outcome displeases us now or later, we sue. It's the thing to do. Every day armies of lawyers and their satisfied clients fill thousands of minutes of airtime telling us that we should sue. That's their solution to errors: sue. It's our just reward, right? After all, medicine isn't supposed to be risky. It's supposed to be a sure thing— zero failure rate.

As we've seen, med-mal lawsuits lead to big settlements, higher insurance costs for doctors and patients, and enough excess testing to drive anyone crazy. How can this happen? It's easy when our courts create precedents putting the force of law behind the ideal of perfection. Why do courts create these precedents? Because we ask them to. We see the TV ads, hire the lawyers, and seek our rewards from judges and juries. The judges, juries, lawyers, and plaintiffs all buy into standards that require perfection. We all want perfection; and we all know that something is wrong.

Some Americans want a government takeover, while others advocate a private enterprise approach free of all public meddling. Whenever we debate national healthcare issues, these two sides stake out their extreme positions.

They frame every detail in the language of Armageddon, polarizing attitudes, while they guarantee the status quo.

We might see this as inevitable. Health is our most important commodity. It defines the way we look at the world. When one's health is good, life is good. If one is in constant pain or discomfort, life is bad. Our health is our key to love, learning, happiness and longevity. It's the difference between being happy and being sad. It plays on our emotions, both positive and negative. We all want long, healthy lives. Not all of us can have them. That's the starkest reminder of our inequality: Some of us will live in pleasure, while others live in pain. Some will live a century, some won't make it through childhood. Health is not justice. Health is not fair. Health is not ethical, moral or wise. Health is health.

The main tool of the extremists on both sides is fear. Those who want socialized medicine play on fears of poverty and bankruptcy. Those who demand the end of all public sector health measures exploit fears of rationing, death panels, and stifling regulations. Neither side makes sense, nor do most of the voices in the middle. They are like the multiple tongues of Babel—incomprehensible. The common thread in all their arguments is confusion. As long as people are trying to fix the existing "system" that will be true.

The cliché we apply to almost every problem is that the solution lies in education. Cliché or not, it's certainly true of healthcare. We all need education, including refresher courses in logic, finance, and math. But more than that, we have to learn how to take responsibility for ourselves, and how to set limits.

We must start with ourselves. Each of us must begin with the questions: What do I want from my healthcare providers? What can I realistically expect from them? For most of us the answer to the first question is the same thing I noted above: we want it all. To state it plainly: we want to live as well as we can for as long as we can. If we think of it that way, we might start making sense. We can never have it all, but we can usually have it better. How?

The first place to apply realistic principles is in our attitude toward procedures and treatments. We must accept the fact that there is always risk. We must see that a zero failure rate is more myth than goal. Even when we do all the right things, we make mistakes. After all, we're human. We then must extend this acceptance of risk to our machines, drugs, and health-related systems. Our fellow humans devise and operate these things, so the devices are as likely to fail as we are. This doesn't mean we have to tolerate negligence or incompetence. It simply means we have to expect honest mistakes and inevitable glitches even when competent caregivers are doing their best.

Next, we must wean ourselves from our current "system" of health insurance. That's not to say that insurance doesn't have a role in the economics of healthcare, but it should be insurance in the old sense of that word. It should insure you against things that you hope won't happen at all. If we can foresee we'll need money for a specific necessity, we put the funds aside. That's how we deal with our normal budget concerns. If we know unexpected calamities can come out of the blue, and we want to be sure we can deal with them financially, then we insure ourselves against them. That's what insurance is meant to be.

In healthcare this means that if you need to pay for costly and necessary surgery, intensive therapy, or an available, but expensive drug, insurance makes sense. If you want an annual checkup, it doesn't. Insurance should pay for accidents and catastrophes. Patients should pay for small or elective treatments out of their own pockets. If individuals want to buy medical policies that cover everything down to the band-aids, that's their right, but that shouldn't be a public concern. Any policies covering these elective procedures should be named something other than "insurance." We might call such policies "retainers" or "funds." Either name would indicate that this money could be used whenever we like, for any of our health-centric desires. Insurance would then regain its original meaning. The only insurance you should have to buy is the minimum amount necessary to cover extraordinary and unexpected circumstances. That way, if you get really sick or injured, the rest of us won't have to pay for your irresponsibility. Those who live in poverty would still receive public health funds.

End-of-life circumstances are often unexpected, so insurance will usually cover them. That's fine, but we also need to accept the fact that death is inevitable, and in the end nothing can insure us against it. The immortality of the human body should be seen for what it is: impossible and undesirable. Our bodies aren't meant to last forever. Our attempts to achieve unlimited longevity, and our glorification of that goal, lead to countless brain-dead bodies kept in vegetative states indefinitely. We foot the bill for this horrific treatment every time we pay an insurance premium or a tax bill. We must accept the fact that the human body can't live up to a zero failure rate. Every human body will break down beyond repair eventually. We should do all we can to avoid it, yet we must accept it when it comes.

I always remember the elderly widow I wrote about in the first chapter. When her husband of many decades died, she chose to recall all their happiness, and promise him that she would be with him when her time came. She wasn't cold or detached. She wasn't in denial. Considering her obvious love for her departed husband, I'm sure she had tearful moments later on, but her first impulse was to celebrate the life they'd shared. It was a warmly realistic attitude that provided a perfect ending to their passionate love. If this way of thinking were widespread we could all deal with death more fittingly. Instead we try to postpone our grief by accepting the grim ghost of life lying in a hospital bed. This obscene ritual seldom has any connection to the patient's religious or spiritual beliefs. It usually occurs because our only socially acceptable response to death is resistance. Western culture has never developed traditions for accepting death as a normal process. We don't encourage graceful exits. We should.

So what would a sensible health system look like? For most of our everyday concerns it would be private. Minor matters would be handled at doctor's offices or in private clinics. Minor breaks, lacerations, or other small injuries would be treated and paid for there. Doctors would compete for this business, which would keep prices down. There wouldn't be anywhere near as much paperwork because in most cases insurance wouldn't be a part of the equation. Most policies would cover catastrophes. If a catastrophe occurred the patient would file a claim, or notify his or her insurance agent.

Standards would become more reasonable. Doctors would test for any obvious threat, but would only screen for the most unlikely possibilities at the request of the patient or family. The patient would pay for most extra tests, not the insurance company. Doctors would be obligated to describe sensible options, and patients, or their families would be obligated to make decisions. We should all understand that our choices won't always produce ideal outcomes, and the final outcome for every one of us will be death. This kind of realism would be a driving force in creating a healthcare system dedicated to better lives for all of us. It starts with your next healthcare decision.

Whatever factors go into your next healthcare decision, direct-to-consumer ads should not be a part of it. In a better world DTC advertising of medical practices, institutions, and drugs, would be limited to the Yellow Pages, and print without images or audio. This doesn't have to be required by law; it could be put into the codes of professional organizations like the AMA. Patients could get all the information they wanted on a doctor or drug, but it would be up to the patient to look this up. This is one area where there would be visible alterations beyond the field of medicine. A sensible health system would benefit greatly from the imposition of similar limitations on DTC ads for lawyers. This could be done by the ABA. Let these lawyers say it in print, without any extras. After all, if a lawyer can't persuade you in print, how can you expect her to write a brief good enough to persuade a judge? All of us should remember that First Amendment freedoms of expression are for the readers and listeners as well as the writers and talkers. When our airwaves get clogged with massive sludge buildups of self-interested promotional messages, it breaches our right to reasonable access to information.

The law has a place in medicine. As long as we give members of a profession the training and tools to save lives, the law will have something to say about it. Laws will set standards, and forbid dangerous or destructive techniques. The law will enforce regulations on purity in drugs. The state will oversee licensing of doctors and facilities, and courts will adjudicate disputes, just as they do now. Laws on malpractice should be revamped. Legislators should examine these statutes, and all the court precedents that have grown up around them. They should then rewrite the laws to rationally limit awards, and to discourage frivolous suits, such as those based on unavailable tests or treatments.

Availability will always be an issue as long as new drugs and treatments are being devised. When the first patient gets something brand new, it's virtually inevitable that other patients will be waiting. If the "something new" is complicated and/or experimental, many patients will have to wait quite awhile. That's rationing. It's always been there, and always will be there. Sometimes availability will be a deciding factor in matters of life-or-death. Hard as it is, we must acclimate ourselves to this fact.

"Rationing" does not mean "death panels," but it does mean that potentially life-saving procedures and drugs will be allocated, just as they always have been. Today's rationing "system" makes about as much sense as our healthcare "system." To make this allocation more fair we should develop ethical standards covering it, but, like it or not, economics will play a role. In a general sense, standards should be based on need, but we must also realize that if a procedure is invented at a certain hospital, or a drug is first synthesized in one laboratory, the nearest needy patients will get it first. Inevitably the rich will have an advantage. They have the money to pay for information and travel, so they will be able to hunt down new and limited advances more easily than the rest of us. What we should realize is that, in most cases, the more often a procedure or drug is used, the more common and less costly it becomes.

In a sensible healthcare system doctors will be held accountable to sensible standards. If a doctor abuses, neglects, or otherwise mistreats patients, those patients will have the right to make their case, and receive just compensation. A doctor who's proven to be incompetent will lose his or her license. Negligence and egregious conduct will be fully and fairly judged and punished. Awards to a patient should be based more precisely on actual costs incurred by, and losses suffered by the patient. There should still be awards for pain and suffering, but the standards governing these should be tightened. There should also be better systems of redress for doctors who've been unjustly accused.

In almost all med-mal cases when the defendant doctors lose, they're allowed to keep practicing. If a doctor is still intellectually, physically, and legally fit to treat patients, then any financial judgment against him should not be so high that it would put him out of business, either from payment of the judgment itself, or from the resulting rise in his med-mal insurance premiums. If a doctor acted with malice, or with full knowledge that his neglect or treatment would cause damage, then he should be tried, convicted and receive sentencing. That's technically true now, but with a sensible, ethical healthcare setup, enforcement will be more just. Bodies like New York's OPMC should either be redesigned to function more fairly, or they should be eliminated.

Along with these changes, we should review the state of today's medical ethics. The Hippocratic Oath, and other codes surrounding healing and health, need to be examined in light of modern scientific advances. We need a better understanding of the ethics and morality surrounding end-of-life decisions. As we review laws on malpractice, and public-versus-private funding of controversial procedures, we need to seek an ethical and moral common ground. Medical ethics should be covered more fully in our medical schools. This training should carry over into every doctor's practice. Clinics, hospitals and other medical institutions should subscribe to a common, transparent code governing their actions.

Ideas about legal, ethical, and moral issues in medicine should not be compartmentalized. If a doctor is practicing questionable medicine, isn't it just as questionable for an insurance company to pay for it? If a DTC ad is encouraging irresponsible attitudes about a prescription drug, isn't it just as irresponsible for an intelligent patient to act on that encouragement? Healthcare doesn't fit neatly into a well-defined set of cubbyholes. It's a simmering stew with a thousand ingredients, many with multiple functions. If we're going to make any sense of it, we must approach it honestly, with a clear sense of what's right and what's wrong. That's true of doctors, administrators, insurers, lawyers, and perhaps most of all, patients.

That's right, it all begins with you. You are the patient. You are the one at the center of all these debates. It's your ills that we treat, and your cures that we strive to achieve. I know this as a doctor, but I also know it as a patient. We're all patients here.

As patients we must admit to our own responsibility in the healthcare equation. Once the doctor has left the room, and we're left to our own devices, we must realize that our health is, primarily, our business. If I'm a diabetic, it's up to me to stay away from sugary sweets and alcohol. If my doctor tells me to slow down, and I speed up, I'm the one who causes my heart attack. If she tells me to stop smoking, but I don't, the resulting lung cancer is my fault, not hers.

Responsibility is the key to any successful and humane healthcare system, and it's the primary failing in ours. This is true for every major component. Patients want it all, and healthcare providers want to give it to them. Patients want insurance to cover everything, and insurance companies are more than ready to do it for a price. Capitalists want unbridled medicine-for-profit, while socialists want the government to pay for everything. Obviously some decisions must be made. Just as obviously, no one is making them.

We must consider this responsibility—our responsibility—every time we go to a doctor or healthcare facility. Whenever we overeat, or avoid exercise, we should remember that we might have to pay with extra pounds, added sluggishness, and possibly much worse. We shouldn't limit our freedom to lie on the couch all day eating ice cream, but we should understand that our actions and inactions have consequences.

We should think about this responsibility whenever we see a DTC ad for a prescription drug. Is this something we really need? Or is it the kind of pharmaceutical that might be more at home in a shop that sells sex toys? Will that painkiller get me up and riding my bike again, increasing my chances for good health and longevity? Or will I be felled by one of that long list of side effects? Should I pressure my doctor into complying with my request for the drug? Or would it make more sense to find out what my doctor thinks about it first? Should a doctor agree to write a prescription largely on the DTC-induced request of the patient? Or should the doctor regard such requests in a more skeptical light? Should TV, radio, and other media accept DTC ads? Should drug companies commission them? Should insurance underwriters devise policies to cover everything down to the aspirin? Or should they be more concerned with controlling costs throughout the health industry?

Responsibility, or the lack of it, lies at the heart of thousands of questions like these. If we put all the answers together it's easy to see the problem: few of us want to take responsibility, and even those that do have no way of doing it effectively. How can you change a system that's not really a system?

When we're well enough, but overweight, we know what to do: change our habits. We eat less and better food, and devise our physical fitness regimen. If we make those into habits, we take the weight off, and keep it off. Healthcare is the same way. The only way to make it into a sane, sensible system is to make a habit of doing the right thing.

That's why the beginnings of a sane, productive, and humane healthcare system begin with you and me. Each of us has to start sometimes, which means each of us should start now. The next time you see a DTC ad on TV or in print, do as John Prine once said: "Blow up the TV, throw away the papers." The next time you review your health insurance policy, examine it, and competing policies, with an eye toward finding one that covers calamities, but leaves everyday decisions to you. Even if you have to pay cash for those choices, in the long run you'll be taking back ownership of your health. The next time you go to the doctor, tell her you want to make the sanest, most sensible decisions possible about your health, and that of your family.

We all die once, but until then we wake up to life every single day. If each of us bases our healthcare decisions on having the best life possible, eventually those choices will build a better, saner, more life-affirming healthcare system.

APPENDIX I:

SOME FACTS AND FIGURES

As I wrote this book, I came across dozens of books and websites full of statistics. They say statistics can be manipulated to do anything, and recent healthcare debates prove that. Perhaps the best evidence supporting arguments for change can be found in each of our experiences with healthcare. The most pertinent number to you might be this month's insurance bill. Or maybe you've gotten a statement from your provider totaling up the exorbitant cost of Q-tips during a recent procedure. If so, you have your own set of figures proving that our system is out of control. For those who want a little more, here are a few that caught my eye:

- In 1970 total healthcare spending was $75 billion ($356 per person) and represented 7.2% of the GDP.

- Since 1970, healthcare spending has grown at an average annual rate of 9.6% (2.4% faster than the rest of the economy).

- In 2010 total healthcare spending in the United States was $2.6 trillion (about $8,400 per person). It is projected to rise to $4.2 trillion by 2016 (20% of GDP).

- In 2007, the average premium for an employer health plan for a family of four was close to $12,100.

- In 2010 spending for personal healthcare reached $22 billion. Public and private insurance paid $19 billion of this. Not quite $3 billion, or less than 1/7 was paid out of pocket.

- In 2009 the average insured family paid $1,017 per year to cover those who are uninsured (part of our "rob from the rich to pay for the poor" financing system).

- Spending on healthcare takes up more of consumers' income than housing, food or clothing (as a percentage of disposable income, 16.6%, 14.4% and 13.1%, respectively).

- Increases in healthcare spending have exceeded the rate of inflation by 2-to-5 times since 2000.

- In 2006, General Motors paid $5.2 billion in medical and insurance bills for its active and retired workers, which added $1,500 to the cost of every car sold. Toyota's costs are $186 per car.

- In 2008 the U.S. spent 15.3% of GDP on healthcare; Canada spent 10.0%, yet Canada has longer life expectancy and a lower infant mortality rate. Despite our higher costs, the U.S. does not provide better quality or access to healthcare relative to many other countries.

The U.S. continues to grossly outspend other industrialized nations on healthcare. In 2009 the per capita total healthcare expenditures for us, and some of the other developed countries were:

- Australia = $2,960

- Austria = $4,289

- Belgium = $3,946

- Canada = $4,363

- Denmark = $4,348

- Finland = $2,546

- Germany = $4,218

- Iceland = $3,538

- Ireland = $3,781

- Italy = $3,137

- Japan = $2,878 (*2008 data*)

- Luxembourg = $4,808

- Netherlands = $4,914

- Norway = $5,352

- Sweden = $3,722

- Switzerland = $5,144

- United Kingdom = $3,487

- United States = $7,960

Most spending on healthcare involves a small fraction of the population. Specifically:

- 1% of the population consumes 21.2% of healthcare spending (averages $41,580)

- 5% of the population consumes 47.7% of healthcare spending (averages $14,601)

- 10% of the population consumes 63.3% of healthcare spending (averages $8,078)

- 15% of the population consumes 73.0% of healthcare spending (averages $5,558)

- 20% of the population consumes 79.8% of healthcare spending (averages $4,029)

- 50% of the population consumes 96.8% of healthcare spending (averages $776)

- The remaining 50% of the population consumes 3.2% of healthcare spending (averages less than $776 per person)

Compare this with our taxes:

- The top 1% of taxpayers paid 39.9% of the total income tax burden (Adjusted Gross Income or AGI = $388,806)

- The top 5% of taxpayers paid 60.1% of the total income tax burden (AGI = $153,542)

- The top 10% of taxpayers paid 70.8% of the total income tax burden (AGI = $108,904)

- The top 25% of taxpayers paid 86.3% of the total income tax burden (AGI = $64,702)

- The top 50% of the taxpayers paid 97.0% of the total income tax burden (AGI = $31,987)

- The bottom 50% of taxpayers paid 3.0% of the total income tax burden (AGI of less than $31,987)

How can we continue to argue with the world about the superiority of American healthcare delivery and quality? The statistics do not support it.

If we just look at the Emergency Dock in isolation from all other facilities, access to healthcare appears to be universal. Anyone can come in, and we have to do something for them. But the uninsured patients arriving for care in the ED are usually sicker because they've waited until their ailment has reached something close to emergency status. These patients require more services than an ED is designed to provide. Our job is simply to deal with the most immediate threats to life and limb, then stabilize the patient. If we can do that, our job is done, and the patient moves on. Once an uninsured patient leaves the ED, he or she is far less likely to have access to follow-up care. These patients' mortality rates are higher than those for the insured. Overall the poor and the uninsured receive fewer tests, fewer interventions, fewer medications or devices. Finally they have fewer successful outcomes.

APPENDIX II

PRIVATE VS. PUBLIC

The biggest issue in paying for healthcare is whether we should pay for it with tax dollars, insurance premiums, or out-of-pocket funds. Often this seems to boil down to a fight over private vs. public. Insurers take the private side, contending that theirs is a free market approach. Supporters of the public approach believe government should play a larger role. Each side tends to paint the other as extreme, and out of step with the will of the people. This argument creates a lot of hot air, empty space, and stasis posing as action. Despite legislation, regulation and court decisions, the fog surrounding America's healthcare policies won't lift. Both sides in the debate ignore the web of contradictions and complications that's grown up, filling the vacuum in between. In this funhouse full of warped mirrors, the public sometimes looks more like the private, and vice versa. It's enough to confuse anyone.

While both sides have their faults, the lesser of the two evils may not be as apparent as either side thinks. America's healthcare system is a mindless stew of both systems, each banging up against the other. Government can't escape many healthcare responsibilities. It must take care of the active Armed Services and veterans. Few would deny health funding for the disabled. At the same time, some of the biggest insurance providers in the private sector get most of their business from plans covering government workers at state and county levels. Many private sector hospitals get government funds, and government health programs draw great benefit from advances made in private laboratories and hospitals. This isn't two cooperative powers joining to achieve the best system possible. It's two ideas adrift in a sea of anarchy. What emerges isn't a system at all.

American healthcare has nothing resembling a free market where competition and price drive quality. Instead medicine is weighed down with vexing policies and contradictory regulations from both public and private sectors. As a result the American consumer looking for healthcare options is caught in a straightjacket. We can't price shop for operations or procedures. Instead we, and our doctors, are limited by our insurance company's reimbursement policy on any particular treatment. The insurer sets the reimbursement rate at a level that makes the most profit, not according to the actual cost of the treatment.

The laws of supply and demand fail in this structure. As more local doctors compete for more patients and visits, they chase more reimbursements, but often less dollars.

Advocates for the private sector argue their approach offers better management and more controls on spending, yet private insurers put 16% of their spending into advertising, billing and ineffective utilization review. The government-funded Medicare system runs on less than 3% administrative operating costs, translating into billions in savings.

We think of individual and employer-paid health insurance as the private sector's way of insuring us against financial cataclysm if we're felled by injury or illness. But is it? More than 50% of bankruptcies in this country result from medical expenses of those who have insurance!

The basic healthcare transaction is no different from any other free exchange. An individual (payer) needs a service; other individuals (providers) supply it. The providers compete for the payer's business. The payer is empowered. This economic function is universal to all industries, including healthcare.

For the system to reform, the structure of reimbursement must change. Insurers and healthcare providers must redesign the healthcare paradigm, making disease prevention, health maintenance and disease education profitable enough to compete with high-remuneration procedures and treatments. Right now the incentives for driving down costs are largely fictional.

Doctors must adapt to practicing low-cost medicine wherever evidence exists of improved outcomes and higher quality. This is not inferior medicine and does not produce a higher rate of substandard outcomes.